Easy & Delicious

# MOCKTAILS

For Every Day

## ALCOHOL-FREE PARTY DRINKS

### FRESH, HEALTHY, EASY TO FIND INGREDIENTS

**Book 1** of the *Mocktails for Every Day* Series

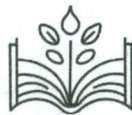

green sauce
PUBLISHING

# TABLE OF CONTENTS

**INTRODUCTION** .................................................. **1**
**THE CLASSICS**
Piña Colada ...................................................... **5**
Virgin Mojito .................................................... **6**
Shirley Temple .................................................. **7**
Cucumber Lemonade ......................................... **8**
Nojito Spritz .................................................... **9**
**SEASONAL FAVORITES**
Autumn Apple Spice ......................................... **11**
Summer Berry Smash ....................................... **12**
Winter Citrus Fizz ............................................ **13**
Harvest Pear & Ginger Cooler ............................ **14**
Spring Lavender Lemonade ................................ **15**
**HERBAL & BOTANICAL**
Grapefruit & Rosemary Spritz ............................ **17**
Basil Lime Cooler ............................................. **18**
Thyme Lemonade ............................................. **19**
Mint & Elderflower Fizz ..................................... **20**
Lavender & Blueberry Crush .............................. **21**
**TROPICAL & EXOTIC**
Mango & Ginger Zinger ..................................... **23**
Passionfruit & Pineapple Cooler ......................... **24**
Guava & Lime Spritz ......................................... **25**
Tropical Hibiscus Punch .................................... **26**
Coconut Lime Refresher .................................... **27**
**FRUITY FIZZY COCKTAILS**
Raspberry Lemon Fizz ....................................... **29**
Peach Basil Sparkler ........................................ **30**
Cranberry Pomegranate Punch .......................... **31**
Pineapple Mint Spritz ....................................... **32**
Grapefruit & Ginger Tonic ................................. **33**

# TABLE OF CONTENTS

## FRAGRANT FLORALS

Chamomile Honey Soother .................................................. 35
Rose Petal Lemonade .................................................. 36
Hibiscus Raspberry Punch .................................................. 37
Violet & Blueberry Breeze .................................................. 38
Jasmine Pear Spritz .................................................. 39

## AROMATIC INFUSION

Lemongrass Ginger Cooler .................................................. 41
Cinnamon & Apple Mule .................................................. 42
Vanilla & Peach Punch .................................................. 43
Spiced Orange Spitz .................................................. 44
Chilli Pineapple Mojito .................................................. 45

## JUST DESSERTS

Strawberry Shortcake Fizz .................................................. 47
Chocolate Mint Cooler .................................................. 48
Berry Cheesecake Spritz .................................................. 49
Caramel Apple Mocktail .................................................. 50
Coconut Cream Pie Cooler .................................................. 51

## TEA-BASED COCKTAILS

Iced Green Tea & Cucumber Cooler .................................................. 53
Early Grey Lemonade .................................................. 54
Matcha Mint Fizz .................................................. 55
Chai Spice Cooler .................................................. 56
Peach Iced Tea Spritz .................................................. 57

## WITH A TWIST

Beetroot & Orange Zest Cooler .................................................. 59
Cucumber Dill Martini .................................................. 60
Carrot Ginger Punch .................................................. 61
Watermelon Basil Smash .................................................. 62
Blueberry Thyme Lemonade .................................................. 63

# TABLE OF CONTENTS

## SYRUPS, INFUSIONS AND CORDIALS

Homemade Grenadine .................................................... 65
Lime Cordial .................................................... 65
Mint Syrup .................................................... 66
Lemon Syrup .................................................... 66
Orange Syrup .................................................... 67
Cinnamon Syrup .................................................... 67
Ginger Syrup .................................................... 68
Basil Syrup .................................................... 68
Lavender Syrup .................................................... 69
Elderflower Cordial .................................................... 69
Cinnamon Infusion .................................................... 70
Rosemary Syrup .................................................... 70
Hibiscus Tea .................................................... 71
Pomegranate Cordial .................................................... 71
Thyme Syrup .................................................... 72
Coconut Syrup .................................................... 72
Violet Syrup .................................................... 73
Lemongrass Syrup .................................................... 73
Rose Syrup .................................................... 74
Honey Syrup .................................................... 74
Chili-infused Syrup .................................................... 75
Chocolate Syrup .................................................... 75
Spiced Clove Syrup .................................................... 76
Vanilla Bean Syrup .................................................... 76
Caramel Syrup .................................................... 77
Dill Infusion .................................................... 77

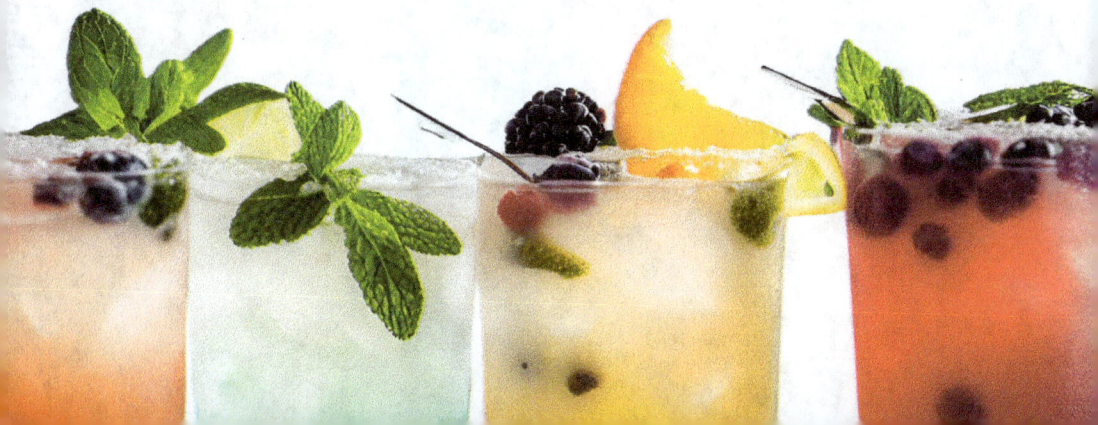

# Welcome to the world of incredible alcohol-free mocktails!

If you're looking for delicious, alcohol-free drinks that are easy to make and even easier to enjoy, you've come to the right place. Easy & Delicious Mocktails for Every Day is your passport to a world of flavor, and it's just the first stop on our exciting journey!

Forget complicated cocktail recipes with hard-to-find ingredients. This book is all about celebrating simple pleasures. We're talking everyday staples, fresh flavors, and easy-to-follow instructions. Whether you're whipping up a refreshing drink after a long day, hosting a party, or simply treating yourself to something special, these recipes are here to inspire and delight, with ingredients you already have on hand or are easy to find at your local grocery store.

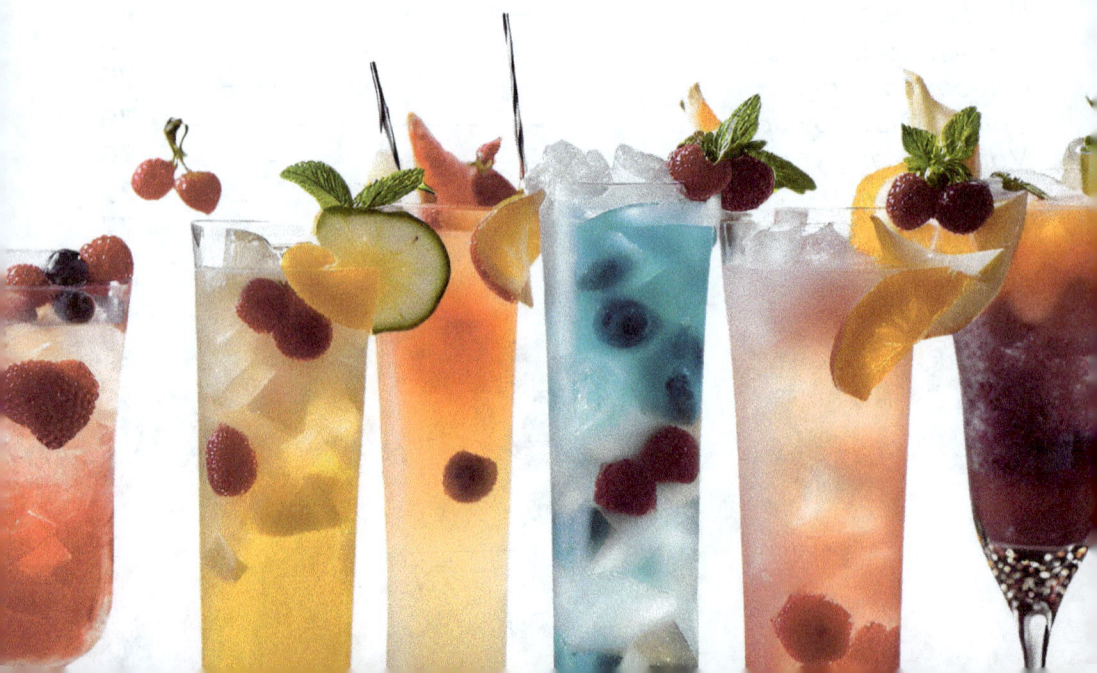

**To get started, you'll need a few basic tools:**

**Pitcher:** For mixing and serving batches of mocktails. Keep it refrigerated for a few hours ahead for colder mocktails.

**Blender or stick blender:** For smooth, creamy drinks and fruit-based blends.

**Citrus press or juicer:** For extracting fresh juice from lemons, limes, grapefruit and oranges.

**Vegetable juicer:** To make vibrant, fresh juices from fruits and vegetables.

**Strainer:** To remove pulp, seeds, or bits of herbs.

**Optional extras for the perfectionist:**

**Cheesecloth or coffee filter:** For an ultra-smooth, refined finish to certain juices or infusions.

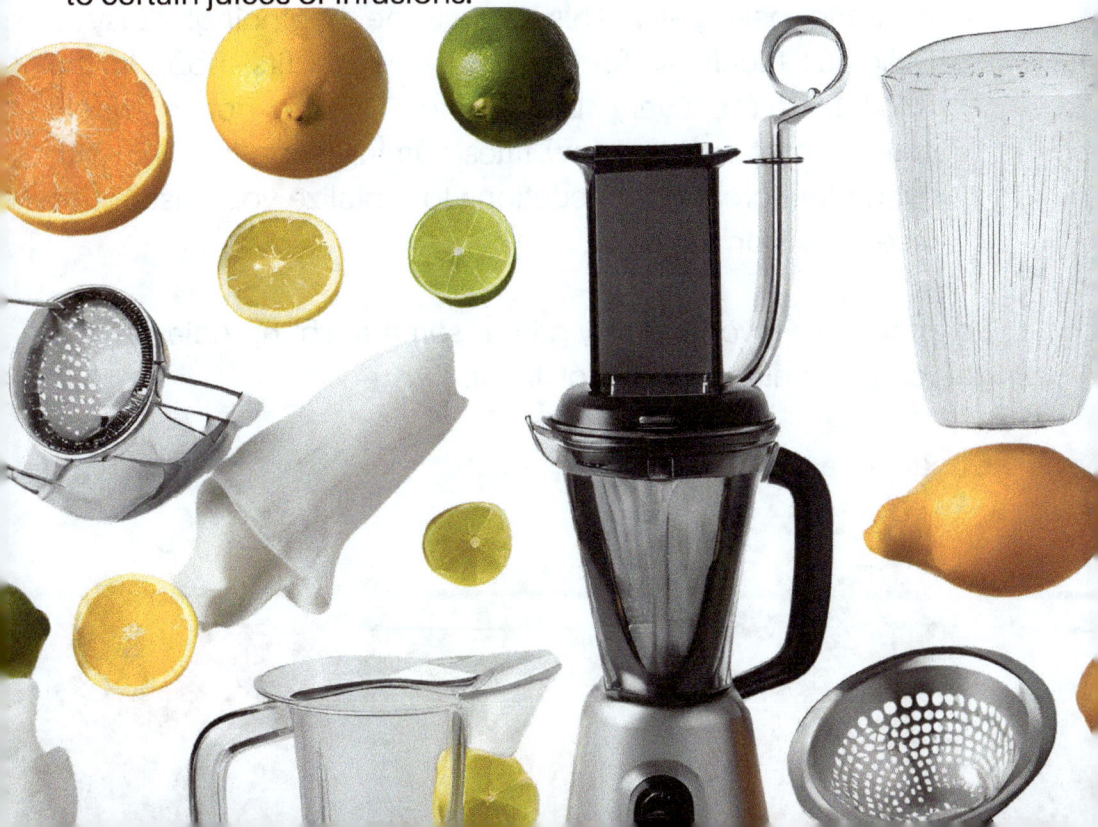

**Inside, you'll discover:**

- Mouthwatering mocktails that are perfect for any occasion, featuring homemade syrups, cordials, and infusions!

- All the mocktail recipes have been designed to make four servings. The syrups, cordials and infusions can be made ahead and will keep for 2-3 weeks in a jar or bottle in the fridge (or freeze them to keep longer and use as ice cubes in the recipes).

- Step-by-step guidance that makes creating delicious drinks a breeze.

- A whole chapter dedicated to making your own syrups, cordials, and infusions – don't worry, it's easier than you think! (Keep an eye out for a dedicated book of in the series coming soon!).

- And the best part? This is just the beginning! "Easy & Delicious Mocktails for Every Day" is the first book in the "Mocktails for Every Day" series. We've got a whole collection of exciting new titles coming soon, packed with even more creative concoctions to tantalize your taste buds (see details on Page 79).

So, grab your favorite glass, gather some fresh ingredients, and get ready to unlock a world of flavor.

**Cheers to a delicious journey ahead!**

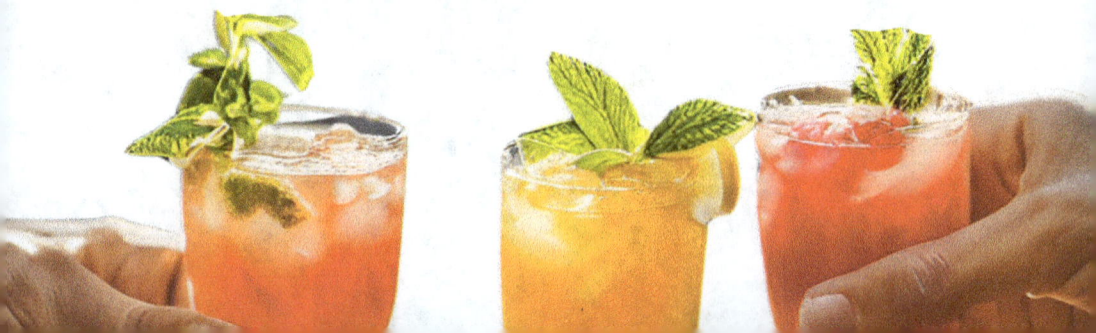

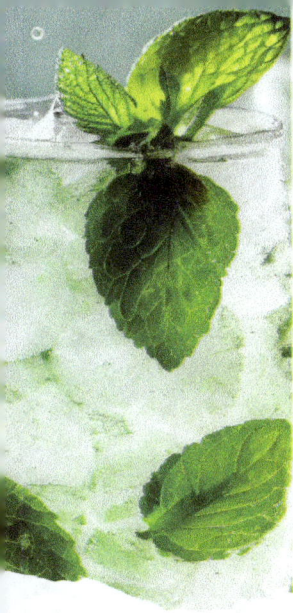

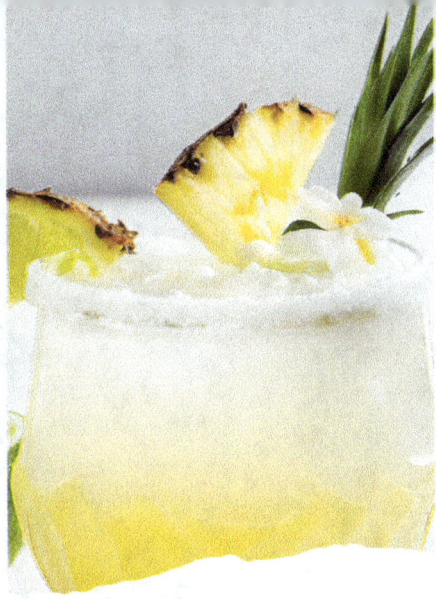

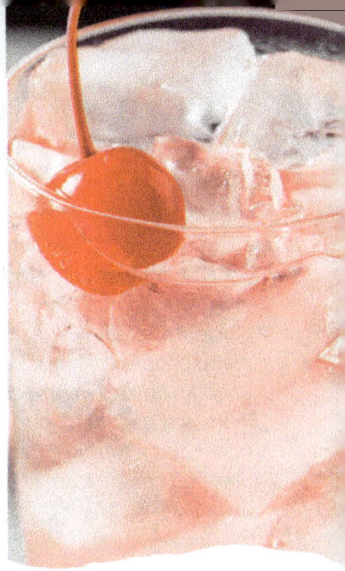

# THE
# CLASSICS

*These classic cocktails with a twist bring fresh, vibrant flavors perfect for any occasion.*

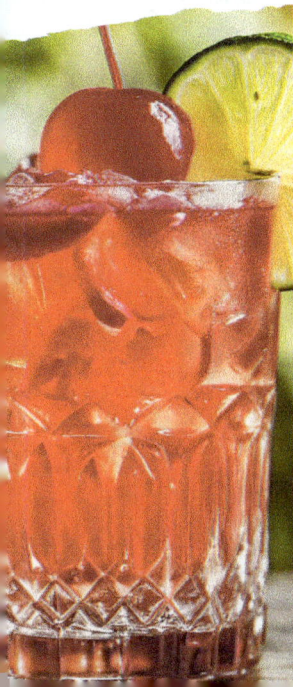

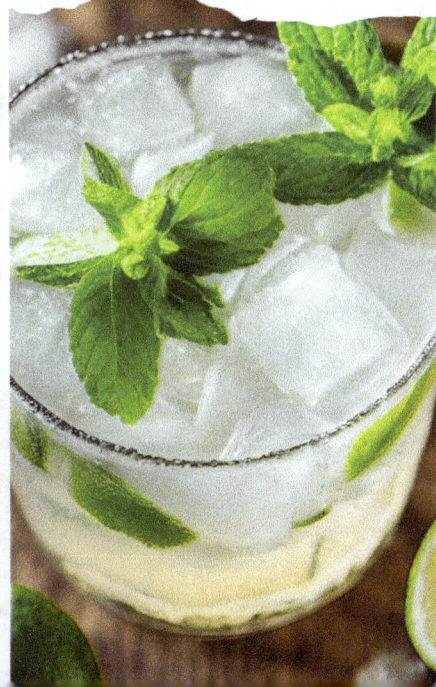

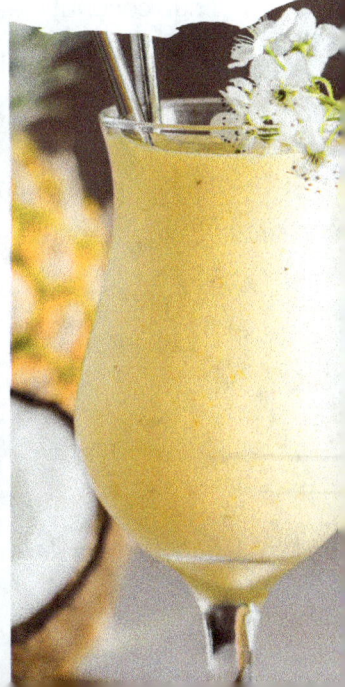

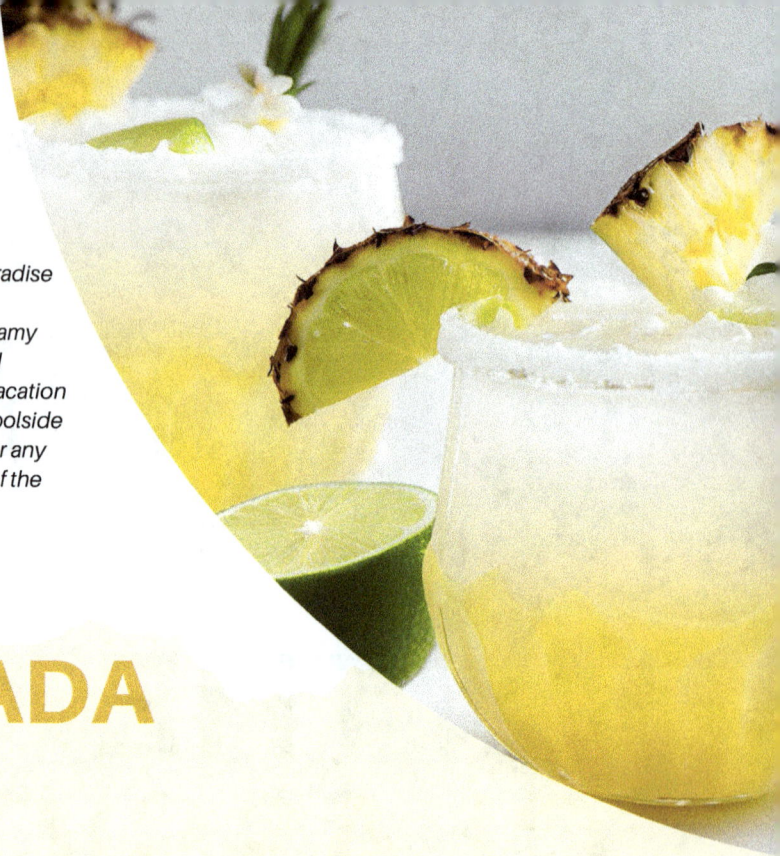

Escape to a tropical paradise with this luscious Piña Colada! Its creamy, dreamy blend of pineapple and coconut is like a mini-vacation in a glass, perfect for poolside parties, lazy Sundays, or any time you crave a taste of the exotic.

# PIÑA COLADA

## Ingredients

- 2 cups fresh pineapple juice (from about 1 small pineapple)
- 1 cup coconut cream
- 1/4 cup fresh lime juice (from about 2 limes)
- Ice cubes
- Pineapple slices and a lime wedge for garnish

## Procedure

1. In a blender, combine the fresh pineapple juice, coconut cream, and lime juice. Blend until smooth.

2. Fill four glasses with ice and pour the mocktail mixture into the glasses.

3. Garnish each glass with a pineapple slice and a lime wedge before serving.

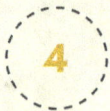

**4**

**SERVING SIZE**

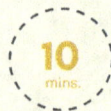

**10** mins.

**SERVING TIME**

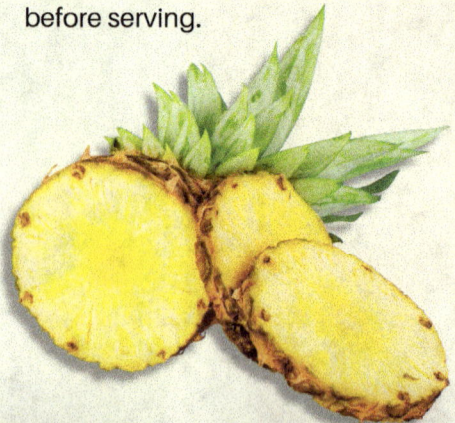

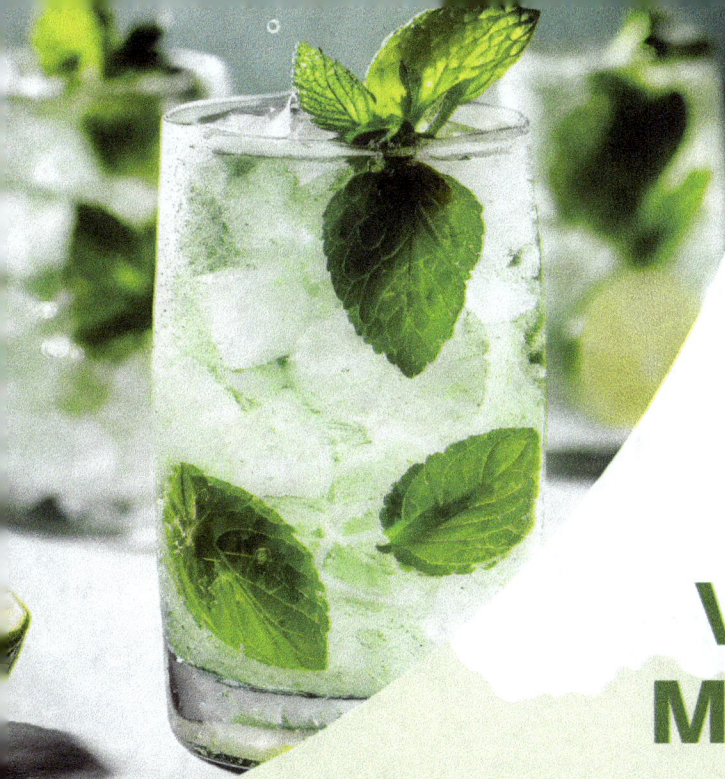

*This Virgin Mojito is a party in a glass! This zesty blend of mint, lime, and sparkling soda is the perfect mocktail to keep you cool and refreshed, whether you're hosting a backyard barbecue, celebrating a special occasion, or simply enjoying a sunny afternoon.*

# VIRGIN MOJITO

## Ingredients

- 2 cups soda water
- 1 cup fresh lime juice (from about 6-8 limes)
- 1/2 cup Mint Syrup (Page 66)
- Fresh mint leaves
- Ice cubes (optional)
- Lime wedges and extra mint leaves for garnish

## Procedure

1. In a pitcher, combine the soda water, fresh lime juice, and mint syrup. Stir well.
2. Fill four glasses with ice (if using) and pour the mocktail mixture into the glasses.
3. Add a few fresh mint leaves to each glass.
4. Garnish with lime wedges and extra mint leaves before serving.

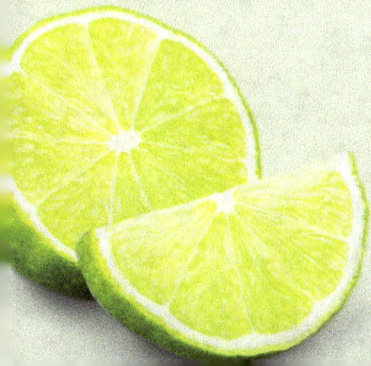

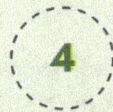

**4**

**SERVING SIZE**

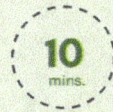

**10** mins.

**SERVING TIME**

*Shirley Temple is a timeless classic that's always ready to party! Its bubbly sweetness and cheerful cherry-red hue make this delightful concoction perfect for birthday celebrations, family gatherings, or any occasion where you want to add a touch of sparkle and fun.*

# SHIRLEY TEMPLE

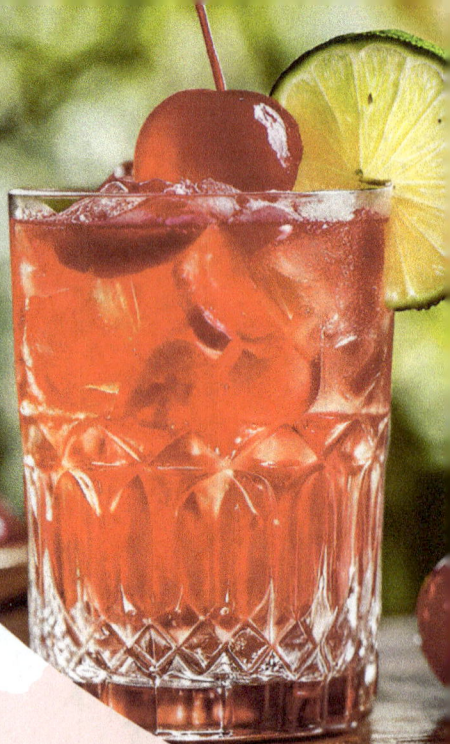

## Ingredients

- 2 cups Homemade Grenadine (Page 65)
- 2 cups lime soda
- Ice cubes
- Maraschino cherries and lime wedges for garnish

## Procedure

1. In a pitcher, combine the grenadine and lime soda. Stir well.

2. Fill four glasses with ice and pour the mocktail mixture into the glasses.

3. Garnish each glass with a maraschino cherry and a lime wedge before serving.

**4**
**SERVING SIZE**

**10** mins.
**SERVING TIME**

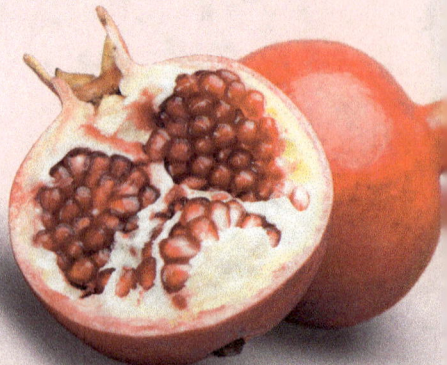

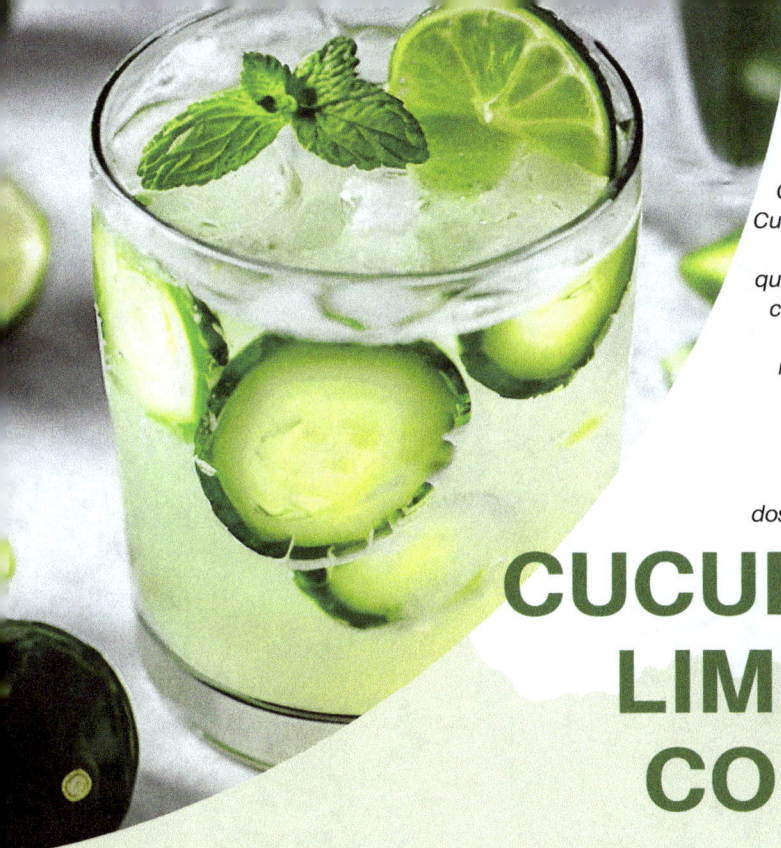

*Cool as a cucumber! The Cucumber Limeade Cooler is an ultimate thirst quencher. The crispness of cucumber and the zing of lime blend into a revitalizing drink that's as refreshing as a dip in the pool. Perfect for a sunny day, a light lunch, or any time you need a healthy dose of delicious hydration.*

# CUCUMBER LIMEADE COOLER

## Ingredients

- 2 cups fresh cucumber juice (from about 2 large cucumbers, pureed and strained)
- 1 cup fresh lime juice (from about 6-8 limes)
- 1/2 cup lLime Cordial (Page 65)
- Ice cubes
- Fresh mint leaves and cucumber slices for garnish

## Procedure

1. In a pitcher, combine the cucumber juice, fresh lime juice, and lime cordial. Stir well.

2. Fill four glasses with ice and pour the mocktail mixture into the glasses.

3. Garnish each glass with cucumber slices and mint leaves before serving

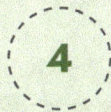

**4**

SERVING SIZE

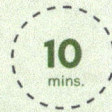

**10** mins.

SERVING TIME

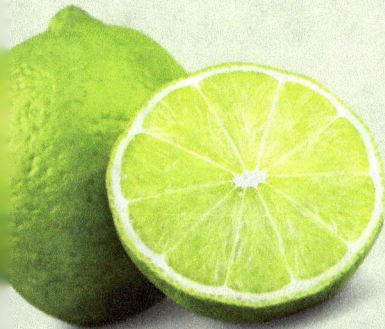

*The Nojito Spritz is your new go-to for sophisticated sipping! This elegant mocktail is the perfect choice for garden parties, brunch with friends, or any occasion where you want to raise a glass to good taste and good company. Cheers to a mocktail that's both classy and refreshing!*

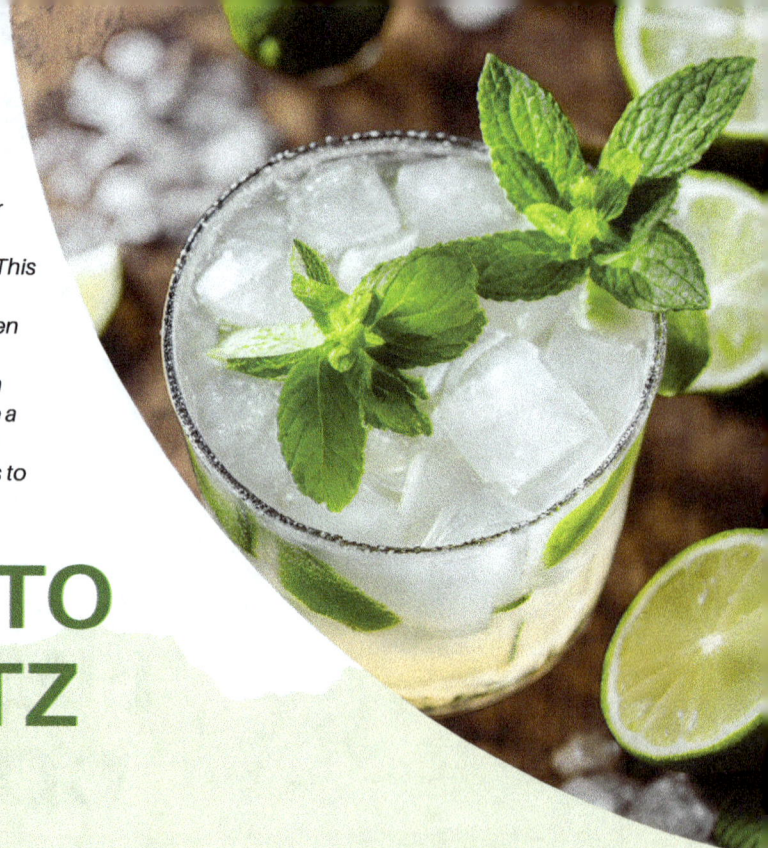

# NOJITO SPRITZ

## Ingredients

- 2 cups soda water
- 1 cup fresh lime juice (from about 6-8 limes)
- 1/2 cup Ginger Syrup (Page 68)
- Fresh mint leaves
- Ice cubes
- Lime wedges and extra mint leaves for garnish

## Procedure

1. In a pitcher, combine the soda water, lime juice, mint leaves and ginger syrup. Stir well.

2. Fill four glasses with ice and pour the mocktail mixture into the glasses.

3. Garnish each glass with lime wedges and extra mint leaves before serving.

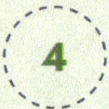

**4**

**SERVING SIZE**

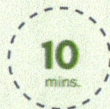

**10** mins.

**SERVING TIME**

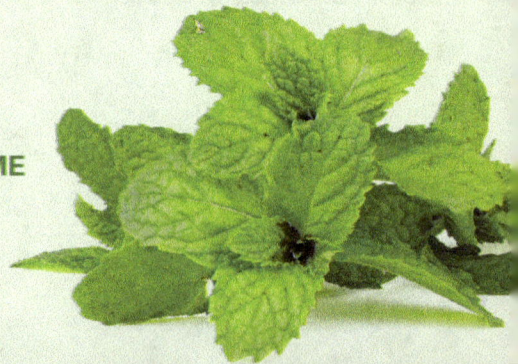

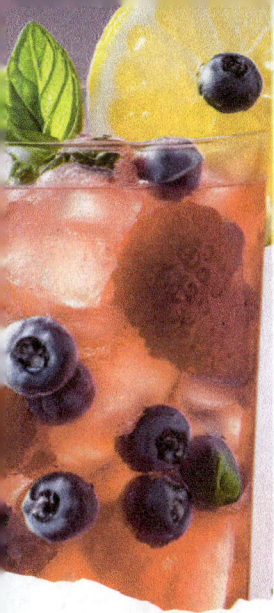

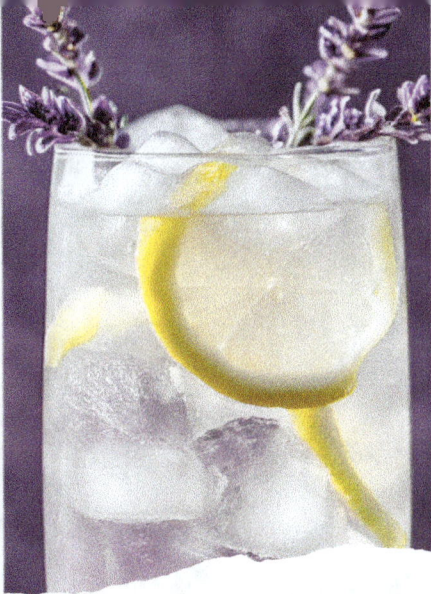

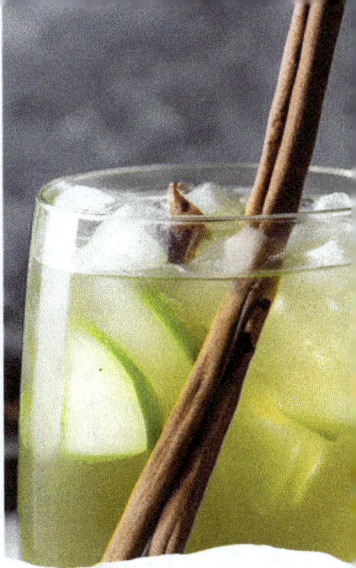

# SEASONAL
# FAVORITES

These seasonal mocktails are designed to capture the flavors of each season, providing a fresh and delightful experience throughout the year.

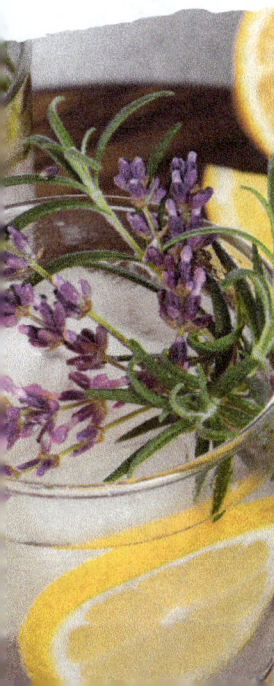

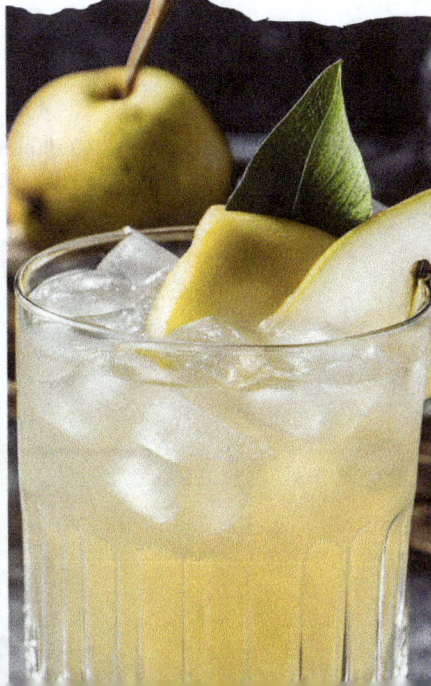

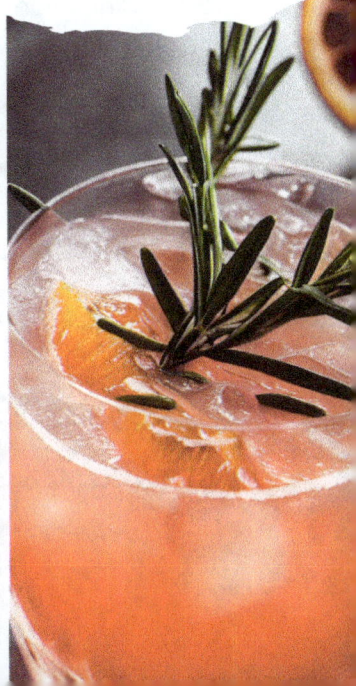

*This cozy Autumn Apple Spice drink evokes the scent of freshly baked apple pie, the comforting spice of cinnamon, and the sweet tang of apple cider, all captured in a single sip. It's the perfect companion for chilly nights, cozy sweaters, and the joy of the fall season.*

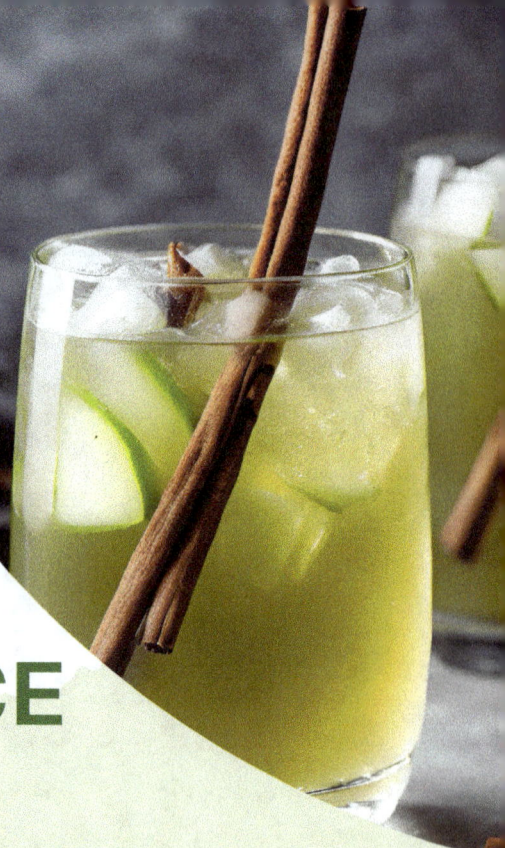

# AUTUMN APPLE SPICE

## Ingredients

- 3 cups fresh apple juice (from about 4-5 apples)
- 1/2 cup Cinnamon Syrup (Page 67)
- 3 cups sparkling water
- Ice cubes
- Cinnamon sticks and apple slices for garnish

## Procedure

1. In a pitcher, combine the fresh apple juice and cinnamon syrup. Stir well.

2. Add the sparkling water and stir gently.

3. Fill four glasses with ice and pour the mocktail mixture into the glasses.

4. Garnish each glass with cinnamon sticks and apple slices before serving

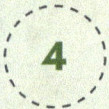

**4**

**SERVING SIZE**

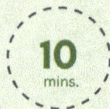

**10**
mins.

**SERVING TIME**

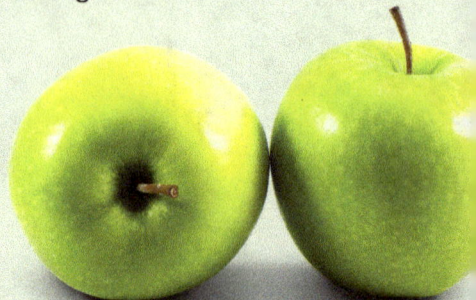

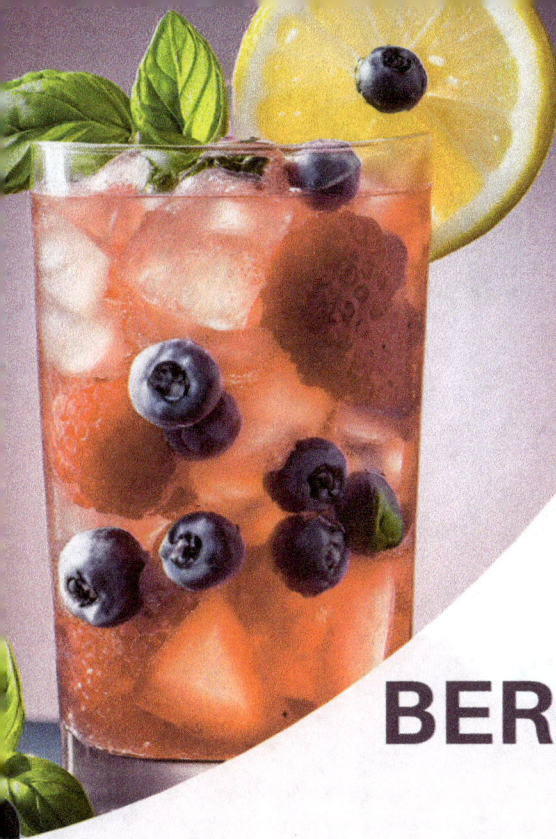

*Bursting with the juicy sweetness of fresh berries, the Summer Berry Smash is the perfect pick-me-up for sunny days. Whether you're lounging by the pool, picnicking in the park, or hosting a backyard barbecue, this refreshing fruity delight is sure to be a crowd-pleaser.*

# SUMMER BERRY SMASH

## Ingredients

- 1 cup mixed berries (strawberries, raspberries and blueberries)
- 1/2 cup Basil Syrup (Page 68)
- 1/2 cup fresh lemon juice (from about 4 lemons)
- 3 cups soda water
- Ice cubes
- Fresh basil leaves and berries for garnish

## Procedure

1. In a blender, puree the mixed berries until smooth. Strain through a fine mesh sieve to remove seeds if desired
2. In a pitcher, combine the berry puree, basil syrup and lemon juice. Stir well.
3. Add the soda water and stir gently.
4. Fill four glasses with ice and pour mocktail mixture into the glasses.
5. Garnish with fresh basil leaves and berries before serving.

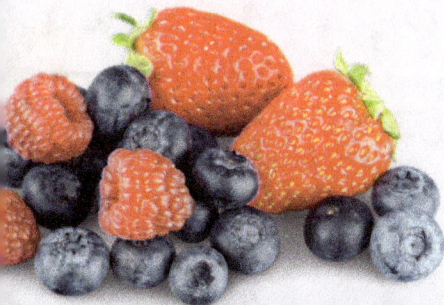

**4**
SERVING SIZE

**10** mins.
SERVING TIME

*This sparkling mocktail is like a burst of sunshine on a cold winter's day. The tang of blood oranges, the invigorating fizz of soda, and a touch of fragrant rosemary that's as delightful as a snowflake. Perfect for holiday gatherings, cozy fireside chats, or ringing in the New Year with a vibrant twist.*

# WINTER CITRUS FIZZ

## Ingredients

- 2 cups fresh blood orange juice (from about 4 blood oranges)
- 1/2 cup Rosemary Syrup (Page70)
- 3 cups tonic water
- Ice cubes
- Fresh rosemary sprigs and blood orange slices for garnish

## Procedure

1. In a pitcher, combine the fresh blood orange juice and rosemary syrup. Stir well.

2. Add the tonic water and stir gently.

3. Fill four glasses with ice and pour the mocktail mixture into the glasses.

4. Garnish each glass with blood orange slices and rosemary sprigs before serving

**4**
SERVING SIZE

**10** mins.
SERVING TIME

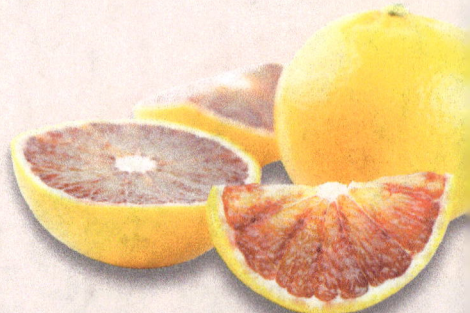

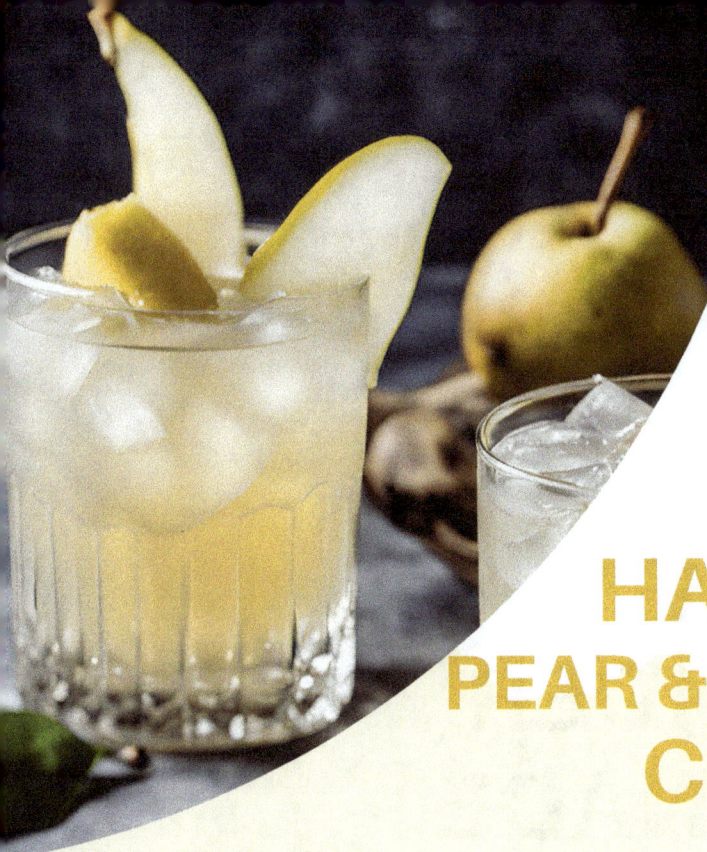

*The gentle sweetness of ripe pears mingling with the spicy warmth of ginger, all wrapped up in a refreshing drink. It's like a cozy autumn hug in a glass, perfect for Thanksgiving feasts, harvest festivals, or simply enjoying the crisp air and colorful leaves.*

# HARVEST PEAR & GINGER COOLER

## Ingredients

- 2 cups fresh pear juice (from about 4 pears, pureed and strained)
- 1/2 cup Ginger Syrup (Page 68)
- 1/4 cup fresh lemon juice (from about 2 lemons)
- 3 cups soda water
- Ice cubes
- Fresh pear and ginger slices for garnish

## Procedure

1. In a pitcher, combine the pear juice, ginger syrup and lemon juice. Stir well.
2. Add the soda water and stir gently.
3. Fill four glasses with ice and pour the mocktail mixture into the glasses.
4. Garnish each glass with fresh slices of pear and ginger before serving.

**4**

SERVING SIZE

**10** mins.

SERVING TIME

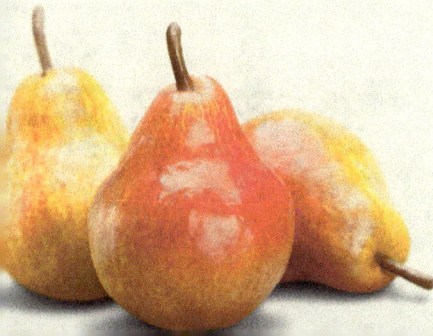

*Spring Lavender Lemonade is bursting with springtime charm. The sweet tang of lemonade infused with the delicate aroma of lavender. is as refreshing as a spring breeze and as pretty as a flower garden. Elegant and perfect for baby showers, garden parties, or any occasion where you want to add a touch of floral magic.*

# SPRING LAVENDER LEMONADE

## Ingredients

- 2 cups fresh lemon juice (from about 8-10 Lemons
- 1/2 cup Lavender Syrup (Page 69)
- 3 cups sparkling water
- Ice cubes
- Fresh lavender sprigs and lemon slices for garnish

## Procedure

1. In a pitcher, combine the fresh lemon juice and lavender syrup. Stir well.
2. Add the sparkling water and stir gently.
3. Fill four glasses with ice and pour the mocktail mixture into the glasses.
4. Garnish each glass with fresh lemon slices and lavender sprigs before serving.

**4**

**SERVING SIZE**

**10** mins.

**SERVING TIME**

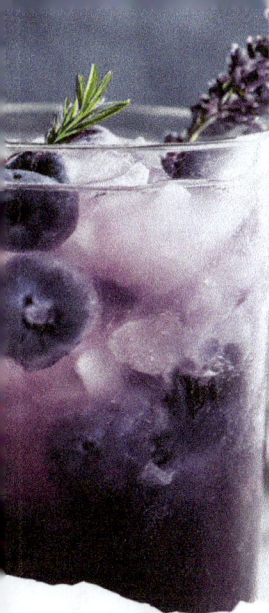

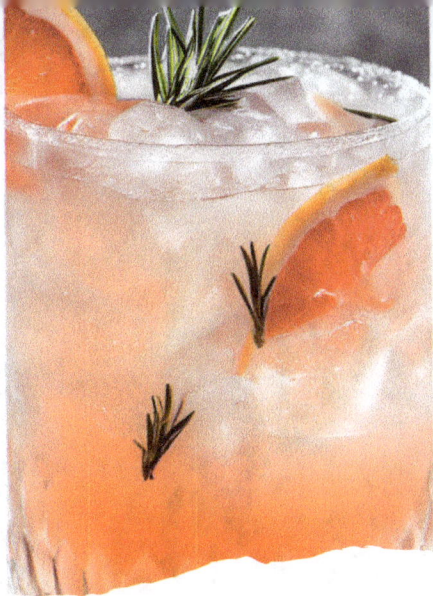

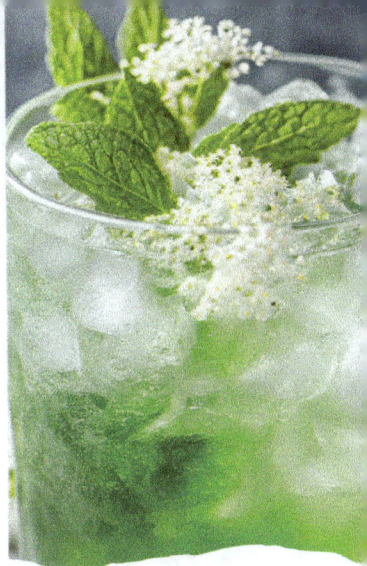

# HERBAL AND BOTANICAL

These herbal and botanical mocktails offer refreshing and aromatic flavors that are perfect for a unique, flavorful experience.

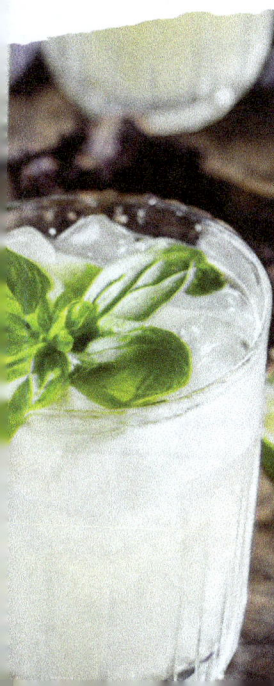

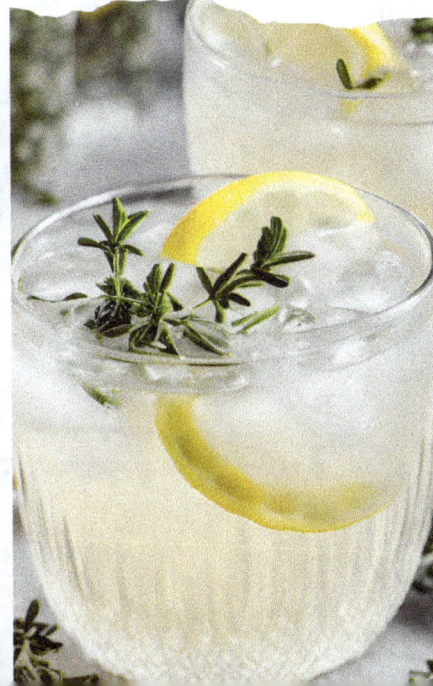

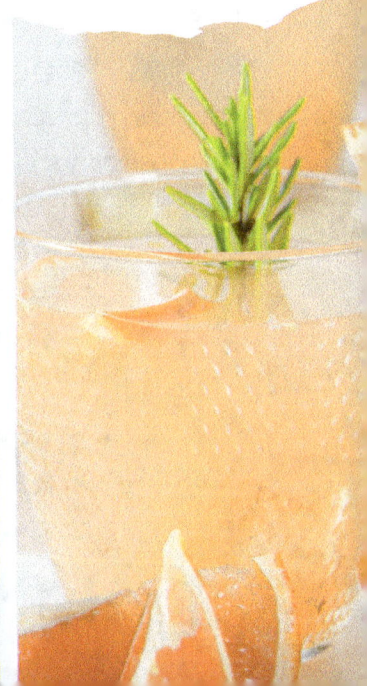

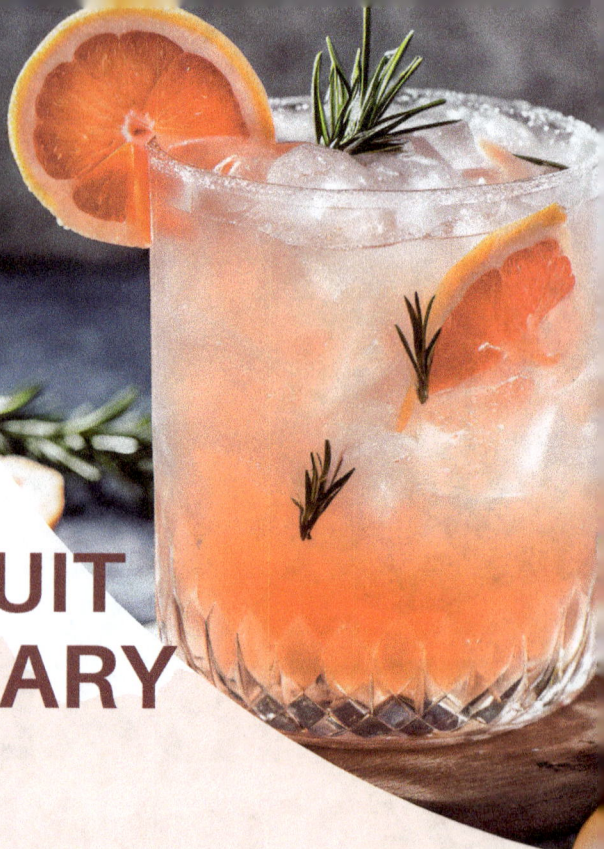

*The tangy burst of grapefruit mingling with the fragrant aroma of rosemary, all brought together with a sparkling fizz. An elegant mocktail that's perfect for brunch with friends, a stylish cocktail party, or any gathering where you want to impress your guests with a touch of refined refreshment.*

# GRAPEFRUIT & ROSEMARY SPRITZ

## Ingredients

- 2 cups fresh grapefruit juice (from about 2 grapefruits)
- 1/2 cup Rosemary Syrup (Page 70)
- 3 cups soda water
- Ice cubes
- Fresh rosemary sprigs and grapfruit slices for garnish

## Procedure

1. In a pitcher, combine the fresh grapefruit juice and rosemary syrup. Stir well.
2. Add the soda water and stir gently.
3. Fill four glasses with ice and pour the mocktail mixture into the glasses.
4. Garnish each glass with grapefruit slices and rosemary sprigs before serving

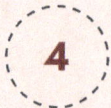

**4**

**SERVING SIZE**

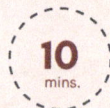

**10** mins.

**SERVING TIME**

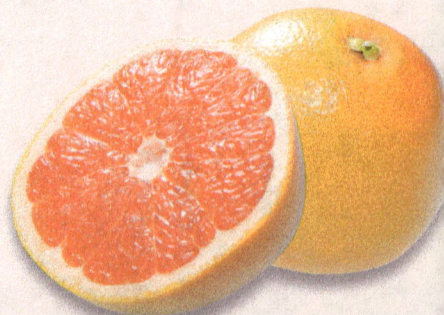

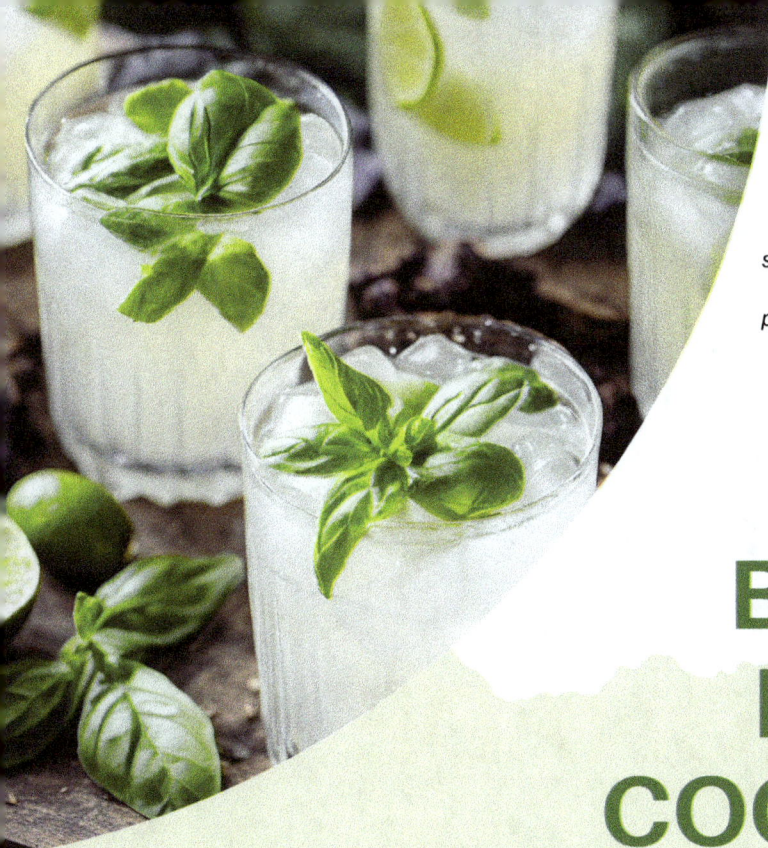

*A taste of summer sophistication! The zesty brightness of lime perfectly balanced by the fragrant notes of basil is like a garden party in a glass. Refreshing and invigorating, perfect for brunch with friends or a relaxing afternoon in the sun.*

# BASIL LIME COOLER

## Ingredients

- 1/2 cup fresh basil leaves
- 1/2 cup fresh lime juice (from about 4 limes).
- 1/2 cup Basil Syrup (Page 68)
- 3 cups soda water
- Ice cubes
- Fresh basil leaves and lime slices for garnish

## Procedure

1. In a pitcher, muddle the fresh basil leaves with a muddler or the back of a spoon to release the aroma.
2. Add the lime juice and basil syrup. Stir well.
3. Add the soda water and stir gently.
4. Fill four glasses with ice and pour the mocktail mixture into the glasses.
5. Garnish with fresh basil leaves and lime slices before serving.

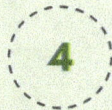

**4**

**SERVING SIZE**

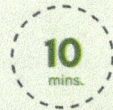

**10** mins.

**SERVING TIME**

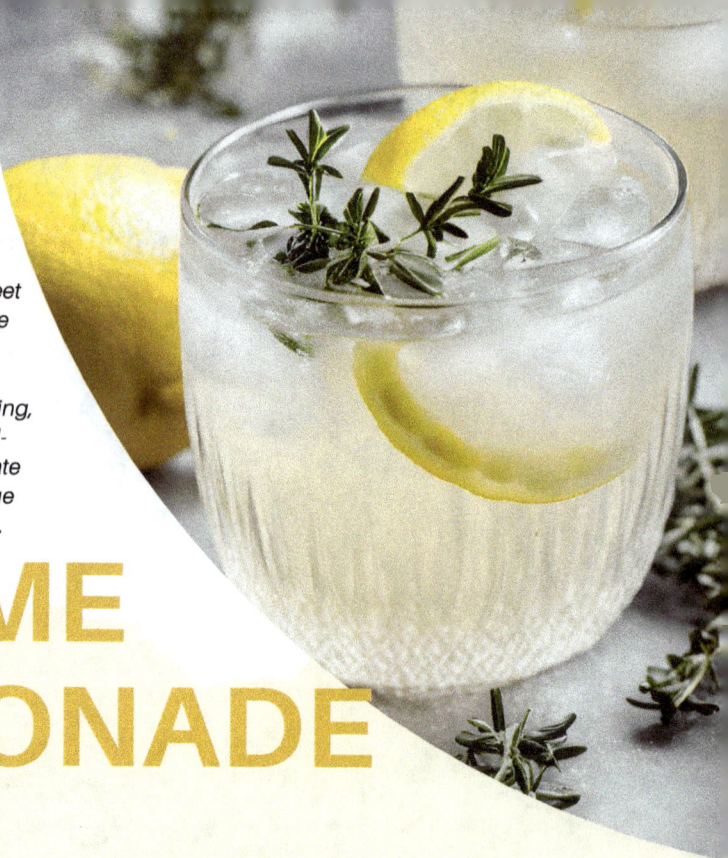

Thyme Lemonade - the sweet and tangy taste of lemonade infused with the subtle earthiness of thyme. Unexpected, refreshing, and oh-so-chic. This herbal-infused lemonade will elevate any gathering with its unique flavor and refreshing charm.

# THYME LEMONADE

## Ingredients

- 1/2 cup Thyme Syrup (Page 72)
- 2 cups fresh lemon juice (from about 6-8 lemons)
- 3 cups water
- 1 tablespoon honey
- Ice cubes
- Fresh thyme sprigs and lemon slices for garnish

## Procedure

1. In a pitcher, combine the thyme infusion, lemon juice, water and honey. Stir well until the honey is fully dissoved.

2. Fill four glasses with ice and pour the mocktail mixture into the glasses.

3. Garnish with fresh thyme sprigs and lemon slices before serving.

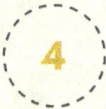

**4**

**SERVING SIZE**

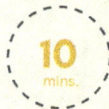

**10** mins.

**SERVING TIME**

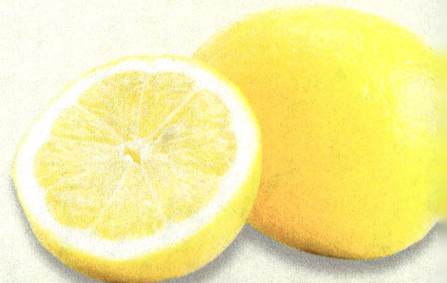

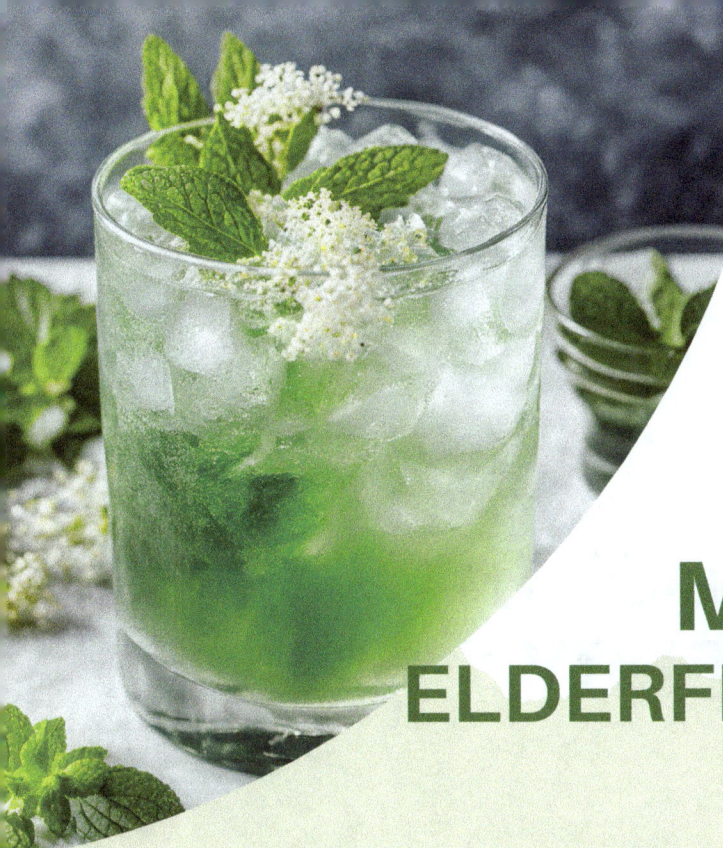

*The delicate elderflower sweetness dancing with the refreshing coolness of mint, all topped with a sparkling fizz. It's a sophisticated mocktail that's perfect for weddings, bridal showers, or any celebration where you want to add a touch of floral magic.*

# MINT & ELDERFLOWER FIZZ

## Ingredients

- 1/2 cup Elderflower Cordial (Page 69)
- 3 cups soda water
- 1/2 cup fresh mint leaves
- Ice cubes
- Fresh mint leaves and edible flowers  for garnish

## Procedure

1. In a pitcher, muddle the fresh mint leaves with a muddler or the back of a spoon.

2. Add the elderflower cordial and soda water. Stir gently.

3. Fill four glasses with ice and pour the mocktail mixture into the glasses.

4. Garnish each glass with fresh mint  and edible flowers before serving.

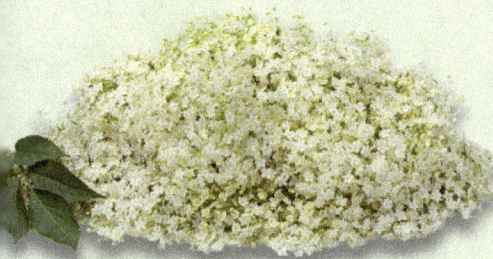

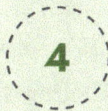

**4**

**SERVING SIZE**

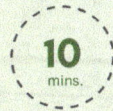

**10** mins.

**SERVING TIME**

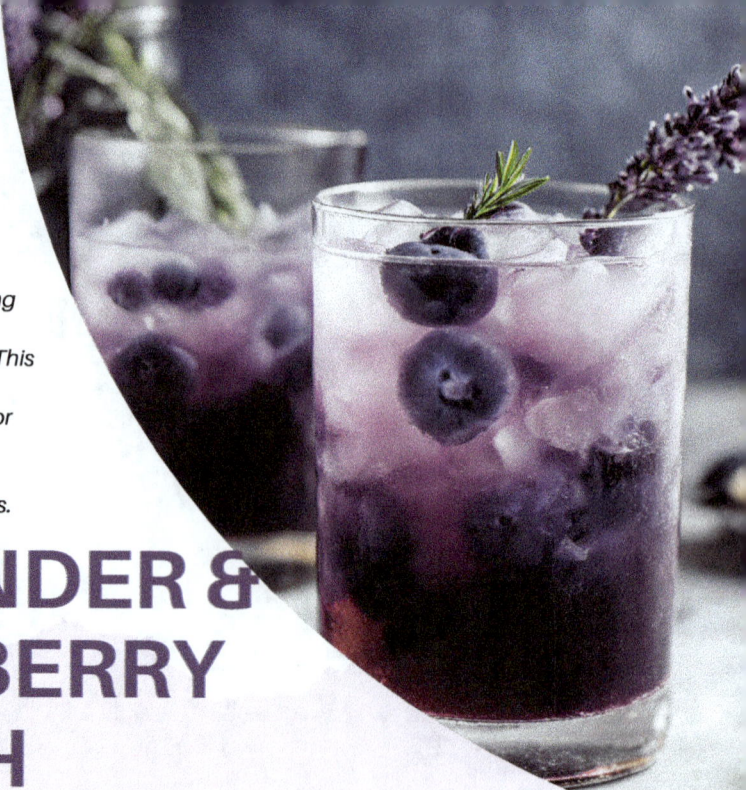

*The indulgent sweet symphony of blueberries mingling with the soothing fragrance of lavender, all combined to perfection. This captivating mocktail is a sensory delight, perfect for garden parties, bridal showers, or intimate gatherings under the stars.*

# LAVENDER & BLUEBERRY CRUSH

## Ingredients

- 1 cup fresh blueberries, pureed and strained
- 1/2 cup Lavender Syrup (Page 69)
- 1/2 cup fresh lemon juice (from about 2 lemons)
- 3 cups soda water
- Ice cubes
- Fresh blueberries and lavender sprigs for garnish

## Procedure

1. In a pitcher, combine the blueberry puree, lavender syrup and lemon juice. Stir well.

2. Add the soda water and stir gently.

3. Fill four glasses with ice and pour the mocktail mixture into the glasses.

4. Garnish each glass with blueberries and lavender sprigs before serving.

**4**

**SERVING SIZE**

**10** mins.

**SERVING TIME**

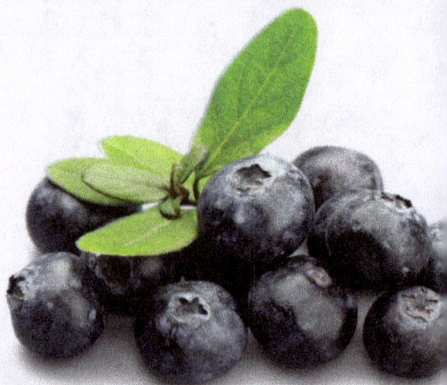

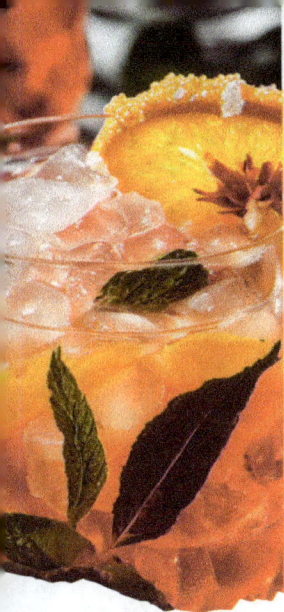

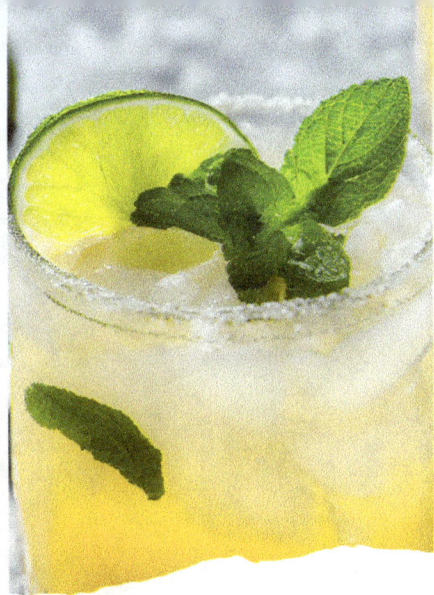

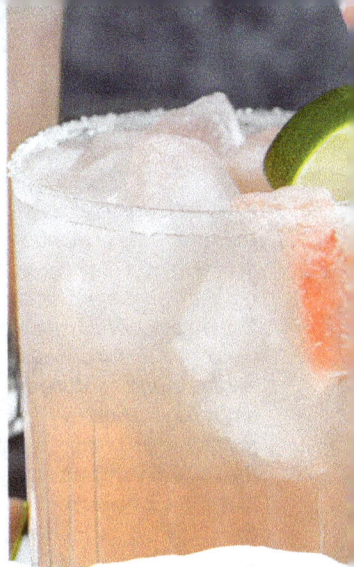

# TROPICAL
# AND EXOTIC

*These tropical and exotic mocktails bring fresh, vibrant flavors that transport you to a beachside paradise.*

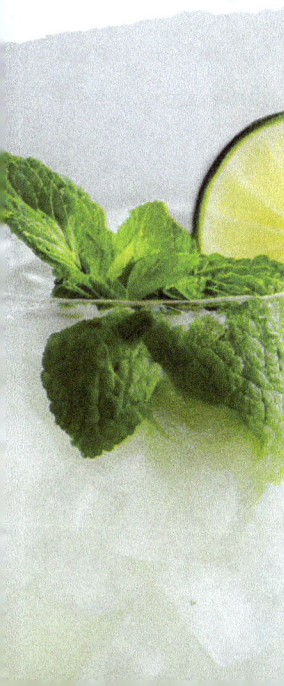

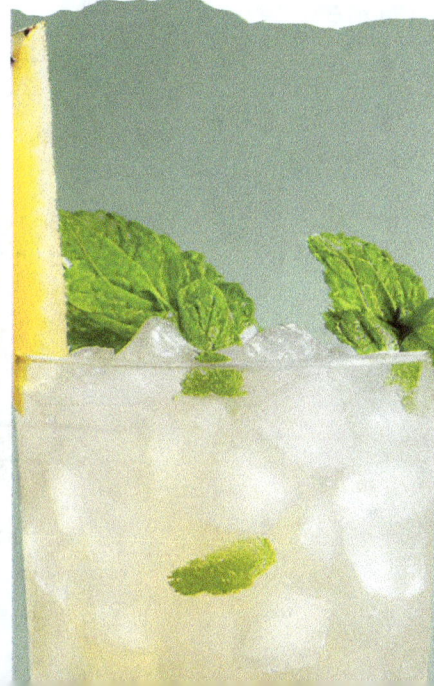

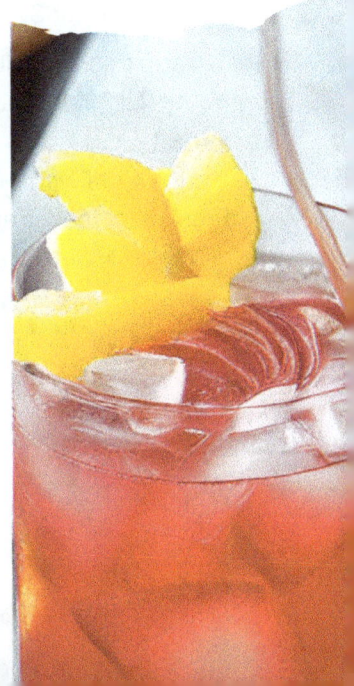

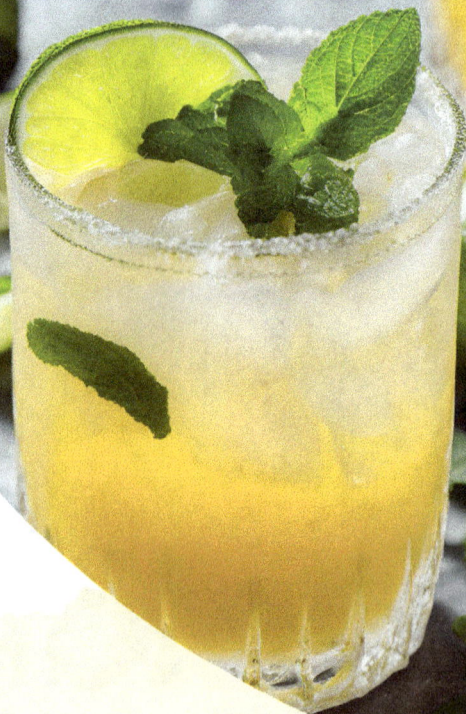

*An explosion of flavor, with the sweetness of mango colliding with the fiery kick of ginger. This vibrant mocktail is like a burst of sunshine in a glass, perfect for poolside parties, summer brunches, or any time you need a revitalizing pick-me-up. Let the zesty flavors transport you to a tropical paradise!*

# MANGO & GINGER ZINGER

## Ingredients

- 2 cups fresh mango puree (from about 2 ripe mangoes)
- 1/2 cup Ginger Syrup (Page 68)
- 1/4 cup fresh lime juice (from about 2 limes)
- Ice cubes
- 3 cups soda water
- Fresh mint leaves and lime wedges for garnish

## Procedure

1. In a pitcher, combine the mango puree, ginger syrup and lime juice. Stir well.
2. Add the soda water and stir gently.
3. Fill four glasses with ice and pour the mocktail mixture into the glasses.
4. Garnish each glass with fresh mint leaves and lime wedges before serving.

**4**
SERVING SIZE

**10** mins.
SERVING TIME

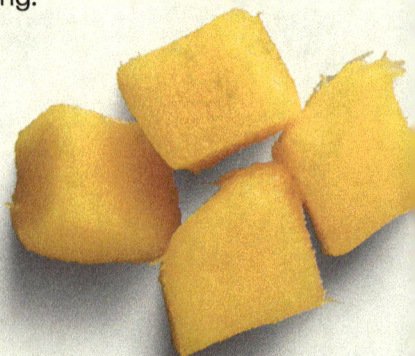

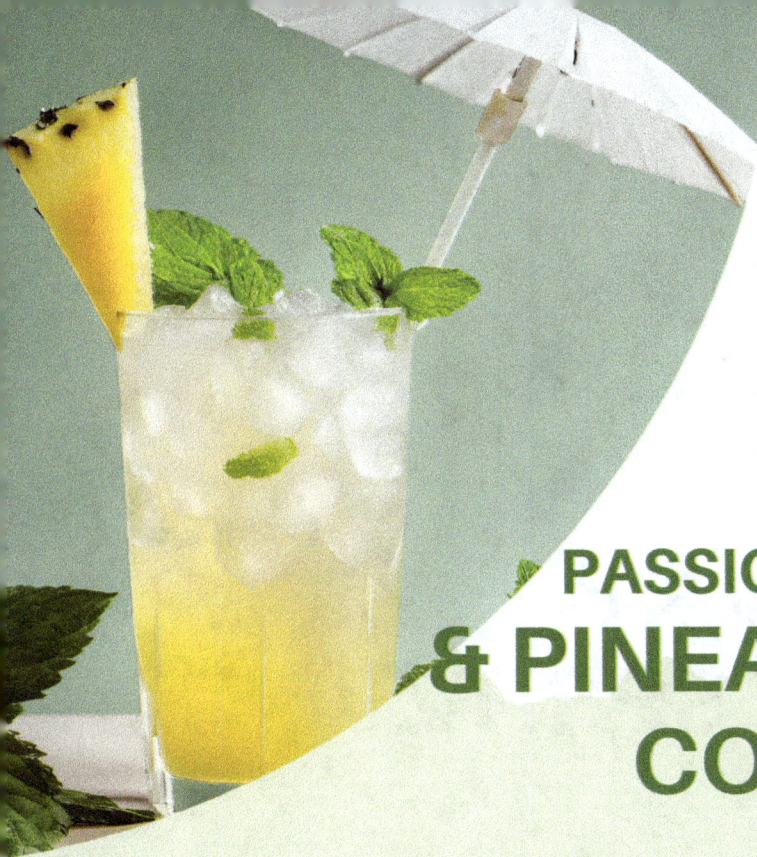

*This vibrant mocktail is a taste of sunshine in a glass, blending the sweet tang of passionfruit with the juicy goodness of pineapple. It's the perfect companion for poolside lounging, beach bonfires, or any occasion where you want to capture the essence of summer.*

# PASSIONFRUIT & PINEAPPLE COOLER

## Ingredients

- 1 cup fresh passionfruit pulp (from about 6 passionfruits)
- 2 cups fresh pineapple juice (from about 1 small pineapple)
- 1/2 cup Coconut Syrup (Page72)
- 3 cups soda water
- Ice cubes
- Fresh mint leaves and pineapple slices for garnish

## Procedure

1. In a pitcher, combine the passionfruit pulp, pineapple juice and coconut syrup. Stir well.
2. Add the soda water and stir gently.
3. Fill four glasses with ice and pour the mocktail mixture into the glasses.
4. Garnish each glass with fresh pineapple slices and mint leaves before serving.

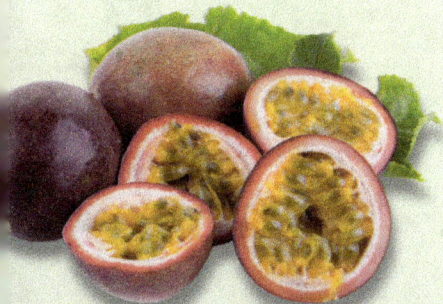

**4**
SERVING SIZE

**10** mins.
SERVING TIME

*A taste of paradise in a glass! Combines the exotic sweetness of guava with the zesty tang of lime, all topped with a refreshing spritz. It's a vibrant and playful mocktail that's perfect for poolside parties, summer gatherings, or lazy brunches.*

# GUAVA & LIME SPRITZ

## Ingredients

- 2 cups fresh guava juice (from about 4 ripe guavas, pureed and strained)
- 1/2 cup Lime Cordial (Page 65)
- 3 cups soda water
- Ice cubes
- Fresh lime wedges and guava slices for garnish.

## Procedure

1. In a pitcher, combine the guava juice and lime cordial. Stir well.
2. Add the soda water and stir gently.
3. Fill four glasses with ice and pour the mocktail mixture into the glasses.
4. Garnish each glass with fresh lime wedges and guava slices before serving.

**4**

**SERVING SIZE**

**10** mins.

**SERVING TIME**

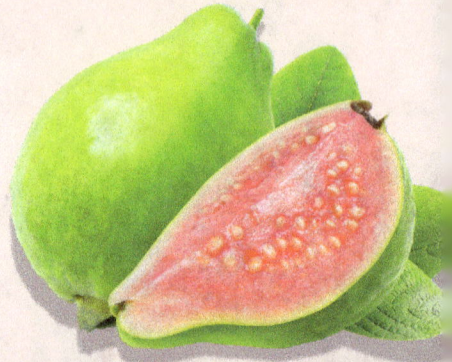

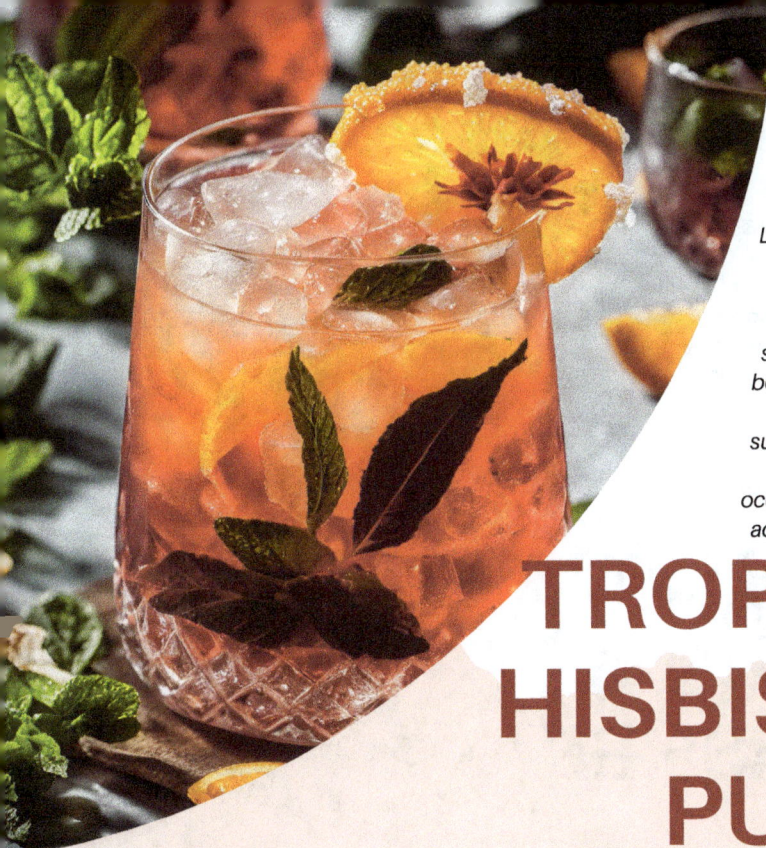

*Like a party in a glass! The vibrant hues of hibiscus flowers mingling with tropical fruits, creating a symphony of flavors that's both refreshing and exotic. A perfect centerpiece for summer gatherings, festive celebrations, or any occasion where you want to add a touch of tropical flair.*

# TROPICAL HISBISCUS PUNCH

## Ingredients

- 2 cups hibiscus tea (brewed from dried hibiscus flowers and cooled)
- 1 cup fresh orange juice (from about 2 oranges)
- 1/2 cup fresh mint leaves
- 3 cups soda water
- Ice cubes
- Fresh orange slices and mint sprigs for garnish

## Procedure

1. In a pitcher, combine the hibiscus tea, fresh orange juice and mint leaves. Stir well.

2. Add the soda water and stir gently.

3. Fill four glasses with ice and pour the mocktail mixture into the glasses.

4. Garnish with fresh orange slices and mint sprigs before serving.

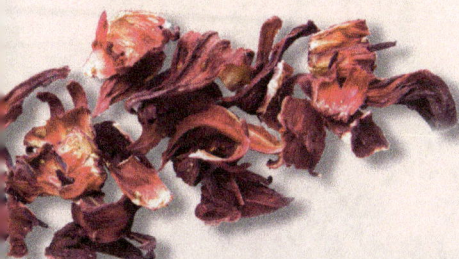

**4**

**SERVING SIZE**

**10** mins.

**SERVING TIME**

*This revitalizing mocktail is like a cool breeze on a hot summer's day, blending the creamy sweetness of coconut with the zesty tang of lime. It's the perfect thirst quencher for poolside lounging, wellness retreats, or any occasion where you want to recharge and refresh with a taste of the tropics.*

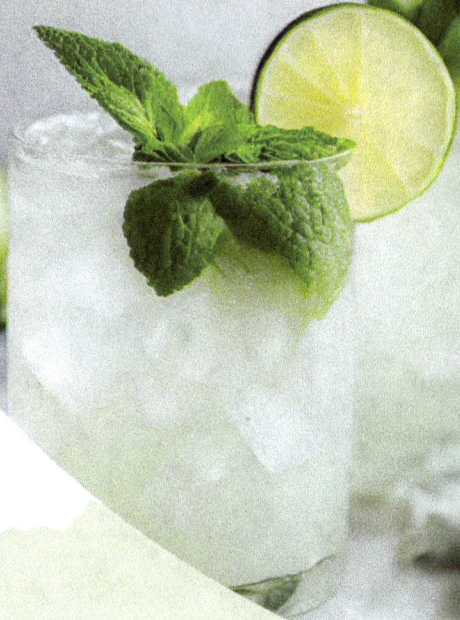

# COCONUT LIME REFRESHER

## Ingredients

- 2 cups coconut water
- 1/2 cup fresh lime juice (from about 4 limes)
- 1/2 cup Mint Syrup (Page 66)
- 3 cups soda water
- Ice cubes
- Fresh mint leaves and lime slices for garnish

## Procedure

1. In a pitcher, combine the coconut water, lime juice and mint syrup. Stir well.
2. Add the soda water and stir gently.
3. Fill four glasses with ice and pour the mocktail mixture into the glasses.
4. Garnish with fresh mint leaves and lime slices before serving.

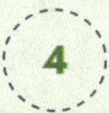

**4**

**SERVING SIZE**

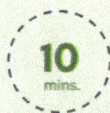

**10** mins.

**SERVING TIME**

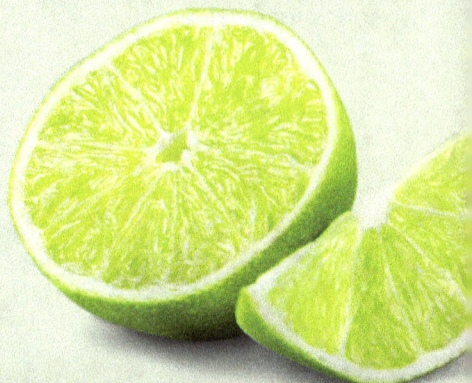

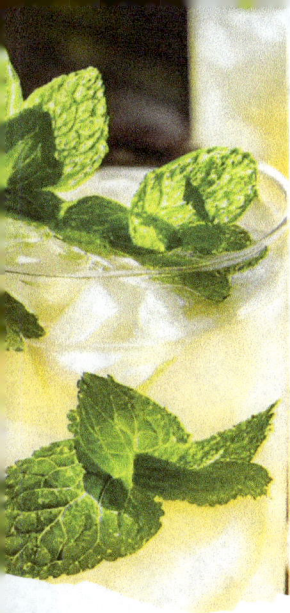

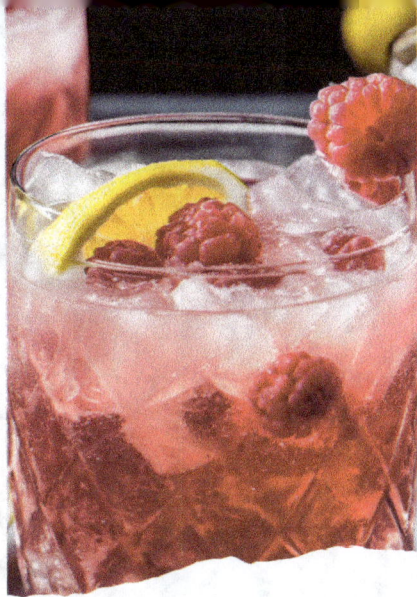

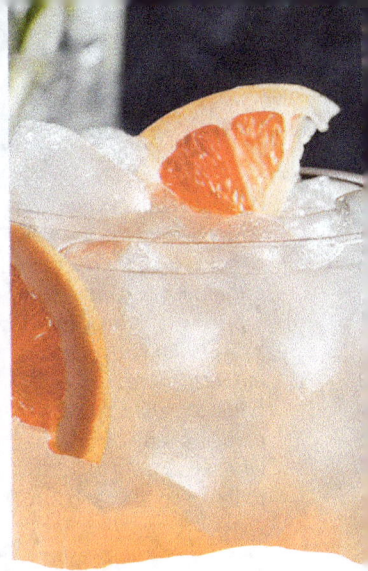

# FRUITY FIZZY
## COCKTAILS

*These fruity fizzy mocktails offer refreshing, vibrant flavors that are perfect for any occasion.*

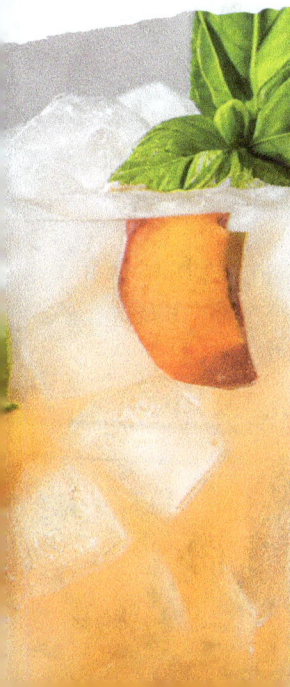

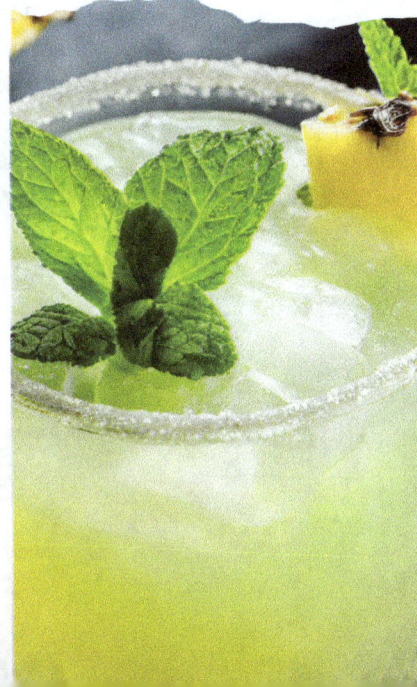

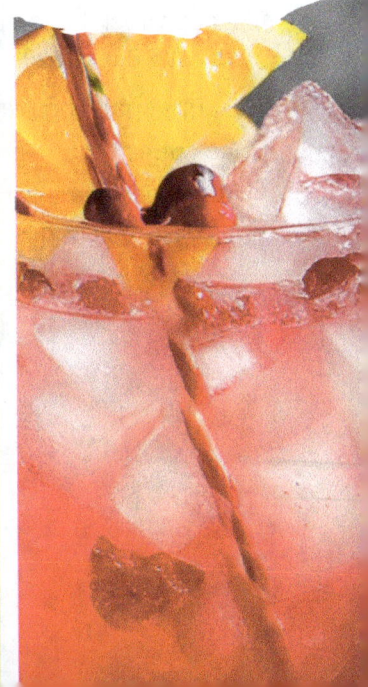

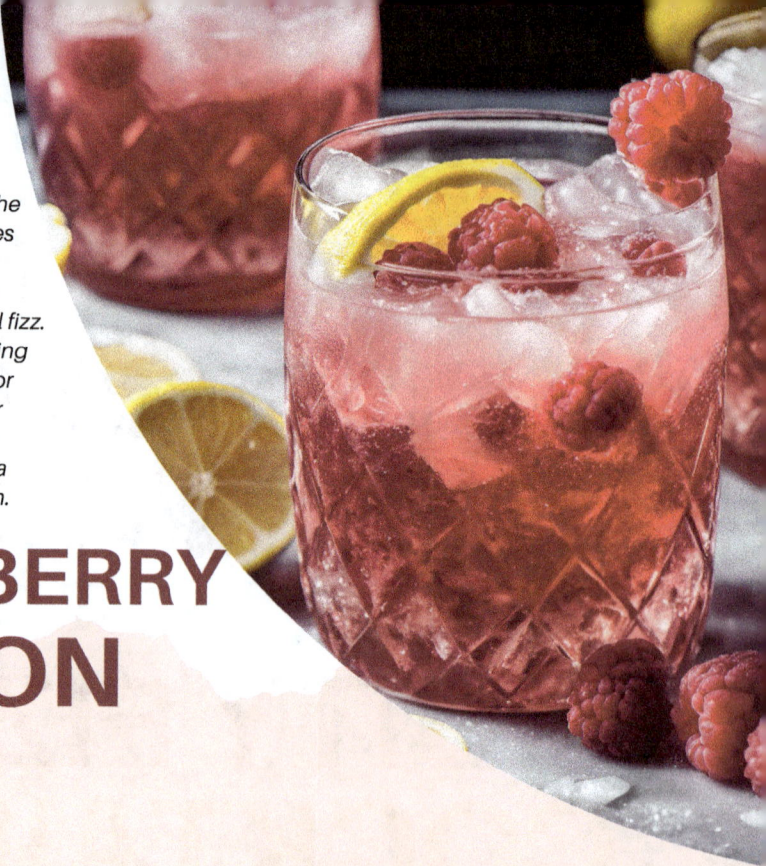

*A burst of bubbly joy! The sweet tang of raspberries dancing with the zesty brightness of lemon, all topped with a delightful fizz. It's a playful and refreshing mocktail that's perfect for bridal showers, summer parties, or any occasion where you want to add a touch of sparkle and fun.*

# RASPBERRY LEMON FIZZ

## Ingredients

- 1 cup fresh raspberries
- 1/2 cup Lemon Syrup (Page 66)
- 2 cups fresh lemon juice (from about 6-8 lemons)
- 3 cups sparkling water
- Ice cubes
- Fresh raspberries and lemon slices for garnish

## Procedure

1. In a pitcher, muddle the fresh raspberries until slightly crushed
2. Add the lemon syrup and fresh lemon juice. Stir well.
3. Add the sparkling water and stir gently.
4. Fill four glasses with ice and pour the mocktail mixture into the glasses.
5. Garnish with fresh raspberries and lemon slices before serving.

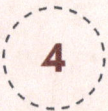

**4**

**SERVING SIZE**

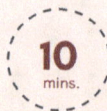

**10** mins.

**SERVING TIME**

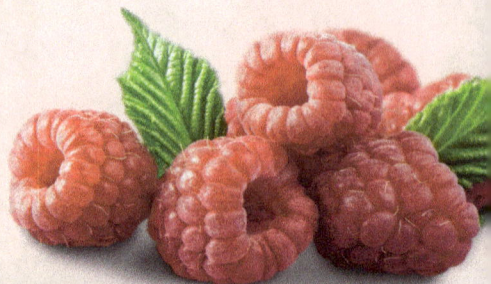

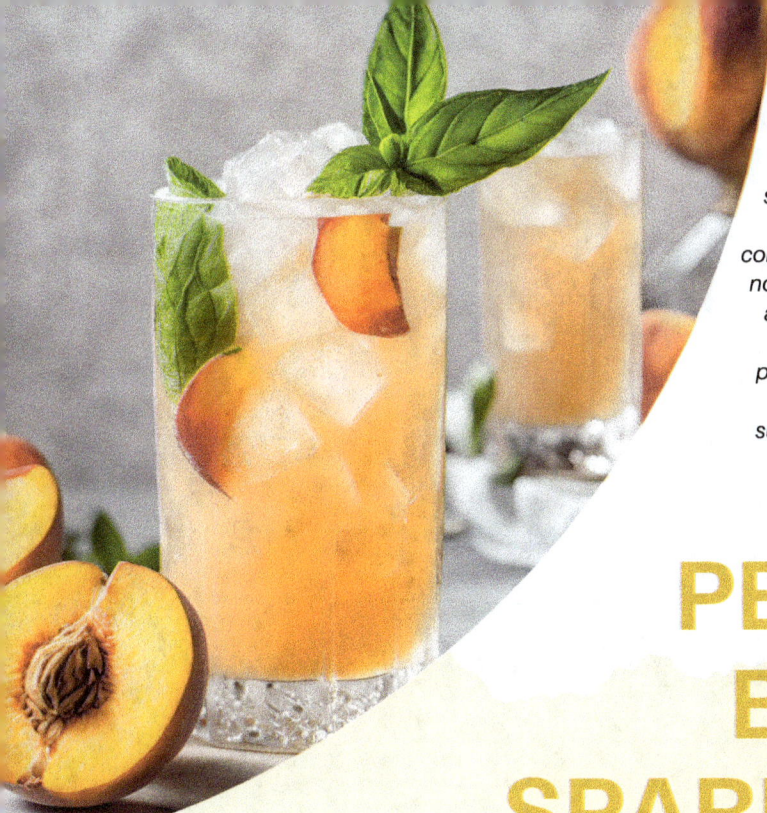

*The epitome of summer sophistication! The juicy sweetness of peaches combined with the fragrant notes of basil, topped with a sparkling fizz. It's a truly elegant mocktail that's perfect for garden parties, bridal showers, or any summer soirée where you want to impress your guests with a touch of refined refreshment.*

# PEACH BASIL SPARKLER

## Ingredients

- 2 cups fresh peach puree (from about 4 ripe peaches, pureed and strained)
- 1/2 cup Basil Syrup (Page 68)
- 3 cups soda water
- Ice cubes
- Fresh basil leaves and peach slices for garnish.

## Procedure

1. In a pitcher, combine the peach puree and basil syrup. Stir well.
2. Add the soda water and stir gently.
3. Fill four glasses with ice and pour the mocktail mixture into the glasses.
4. Garnish with fresh basil leaves and peach slices before serving.

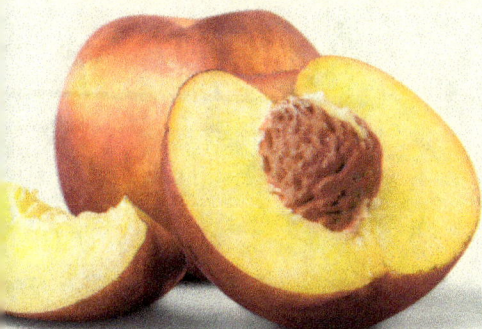

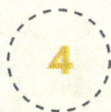

**4**

**SERVING SIZE**

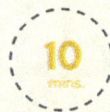

**10** mins.

**SERVING TIME**

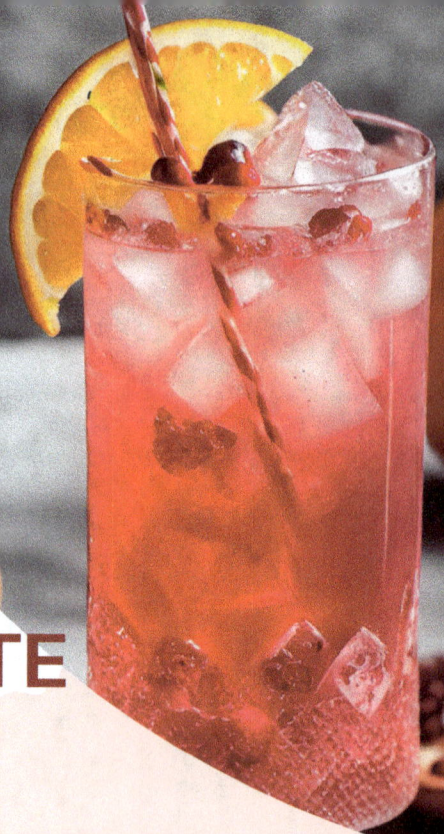

*A festive explosion of flavor! The tartness of cranberries and sweet, tangy pomegranate, creates a vibrant symphony in your mouth. It's the perfect drink to add a touch of holiday cheer to cozy winter parties and elegant brunches. With its rich color and refreshing taste, it's sure to be a crowd-pleaser.*

# CRANBERRY POMEGRANATE PUNCH

## Ingredients

- 1 cup fresh cranberry juice
- 1 cup fresh pomegranate juice (from about 2 large pomegranates)
- 1/2 cup Pomegranate Cordial (Page 71)
- Zest of 1 orange
- 3 cups soda water
- Ice cubes
- Fresh pomegranate seeds and orange slices for garnish

## Procedure

1. In a pitcher, combine the cranberry juice, pomegranate juice, pomegranate cordial and orange zest. Stir well.

2. Add the soda water and stir gently

3. Fill four glasses with ice and pour the mocktail mixture into the glasses.

4. Garnish with fresh pomegranate seeds and orange slices before serving.

**4**
**SERVING SIZE**

**10** mins.
**SERVING TIME**

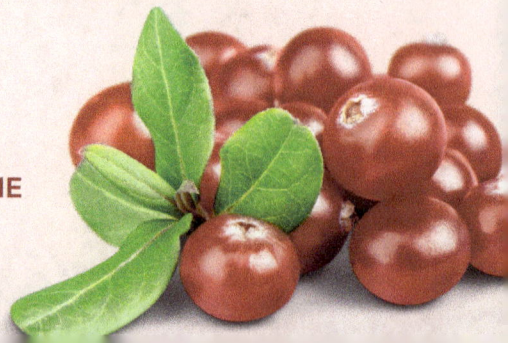

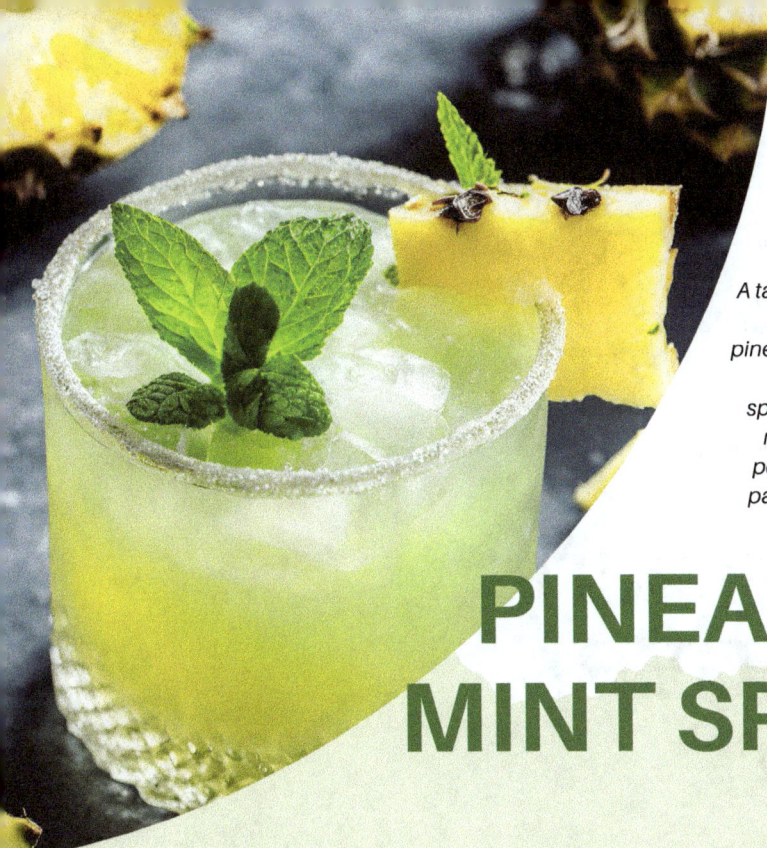

*A taste of paradise in a glass! The juicy sweetness of pineapple and the refreshing coolness of mint, with a sparkling fizz. A vibrant and revitalizing mocktail that's perfect for tropical-themed parties, summer gatherings or lazy brunches.*

# PINEAPPLE MINT SPRITZ

## Ingredients

- 2 cups fresh pineapple juice (from about 1 small pineapple)
- 1/2 cup Mint Syrup (Page 66)
- 3 cups club soda
- Ice cubes
- Fresh mint leaves and pineapple slices for garnish.

## Procedure

1. In a pitcher, combine the pineapple juice and mint syrup. Stir well.
2. Add the club soda and stir gently.
3. Fill four glasses with ice and pour the mocktail mixture into the glasses.
4. Garnish with pineapple slices and fresh mint leaves before serving.

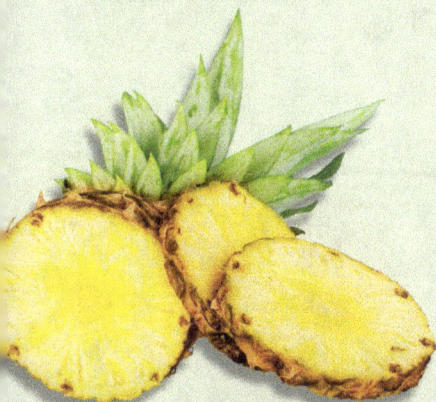

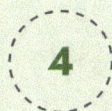

**4**

**SERVING SIZE**

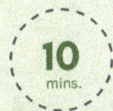

**10**
mins.

**SERVING TIME**

*A tangy burst of grapefruit and the spicy warmth of ginger, create a symphony of flavors that's both refreshing and invigorating. It's a truly elegant mocktail, perfect for dinner parties, stylish brunches, or any gathering where you want to impress your guests with a touch of refined refreshment.*

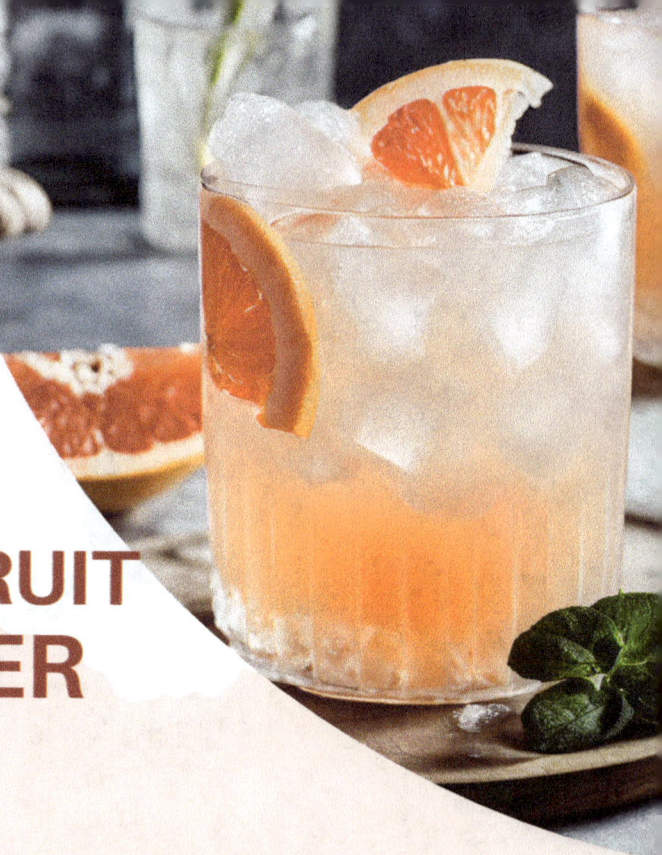

# GRAPEFRUIT & GINGER TONIC

## Ingredients

- 2 cups fresh grapefruit juice (from about 2 large grapefruits
- 1/2 cup Ginger Syrup (Page 68)
- 3 cups tonic water
- Ice cubes
- Fresh grapefruits slices and ginger slices for garnish.

## Procedure

1. In a pitcher, combine the grapefruit juice and ginger syrup. Stir well.
2. Add the tonic water and stir gently.
3. Fill four glasses with ice and pour the mocktail mixture into the glasses.
4. Garnish with fresh grapefruit slices and ginger slices before serving.

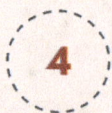

**4**

**SERVING SIZE**

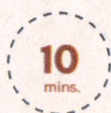

**10** mins.

**SERVING TIME**

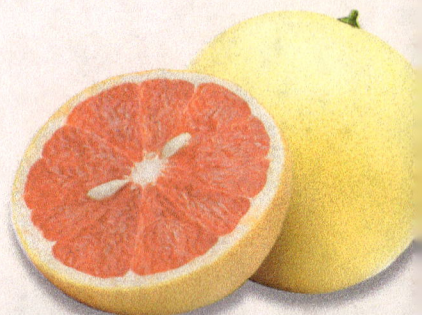

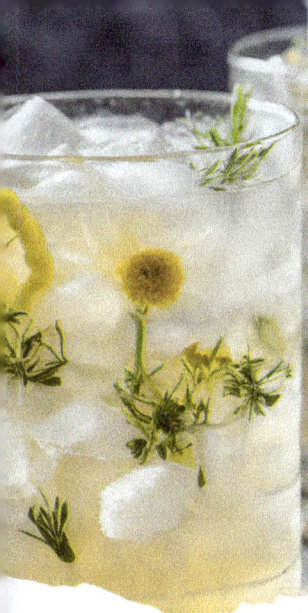

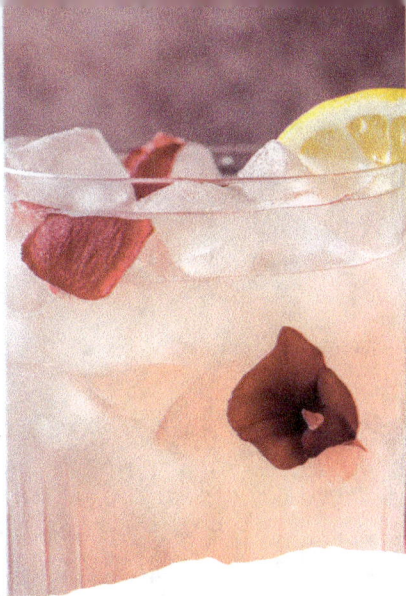

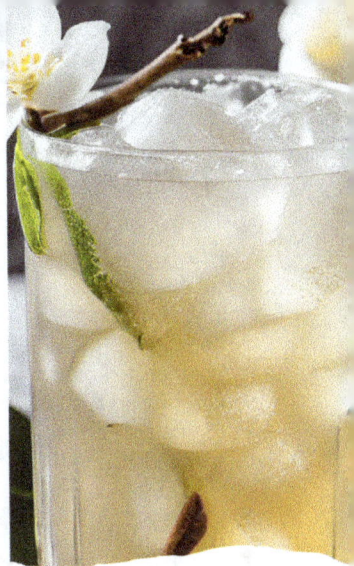

# FRAGRANT
## FLORALS

These floral mocktails are delicate and aromatic, perfect for a sophisticated and refreshing drink experience.

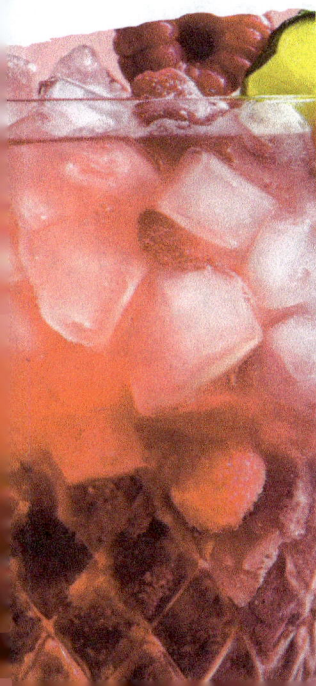

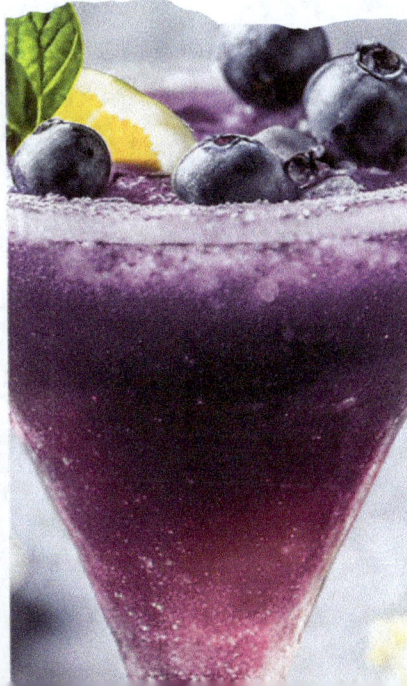

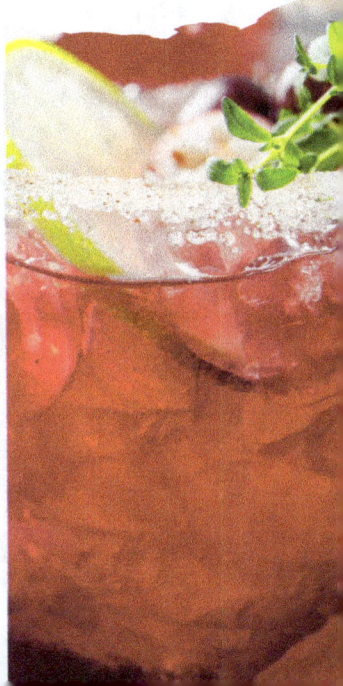

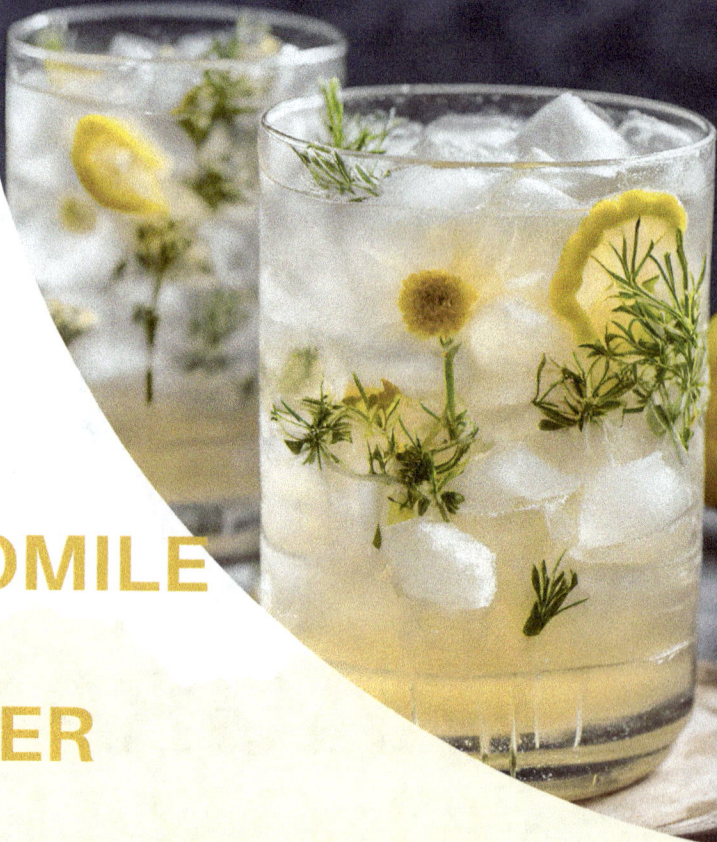

*Soothing chamomile tea with the gentle sweetness of honey. A symphony of comfort and relaxation. The perfect drink to unwind after a long day, to share with friends at a cozy gathering, or to enjoy during a quiet evening of self-care.*

# CHAMOMILE HONEY SOOTHER

## Ingredients

- 2 cups chamomile tea (brewed from 2 chamomile tea bags or 2 tablespoons dried flowers, cooled)
- 1/2 cup Honey Syrup (Page74)
- 1/2 cup fresh lemon juice
- 3 cups soda water
- Ice cubes
- Fresh chamomile flowers and lemon slices for garnish

## Procedure

1. In a pitcher, combine the chamomile tea, honey syrup and lemon juice. Stir well.

2. Add the soda water and stir gently.

3. Fill four glasses with ice and pour the mocktail mixture into the glasses.

4. Garnish each glass with lemon slices and chamomile flowers before serving

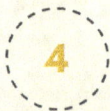

**4**

**SERVING SIZE**

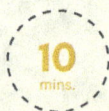

**10** mins.

**SERVING TIME**

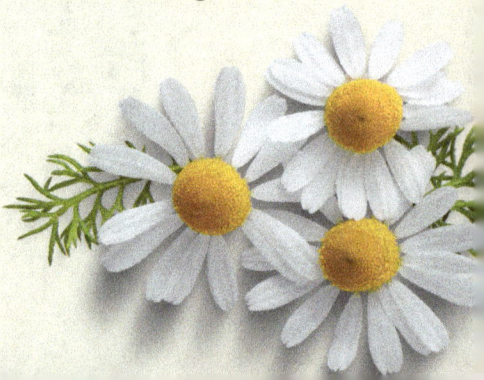

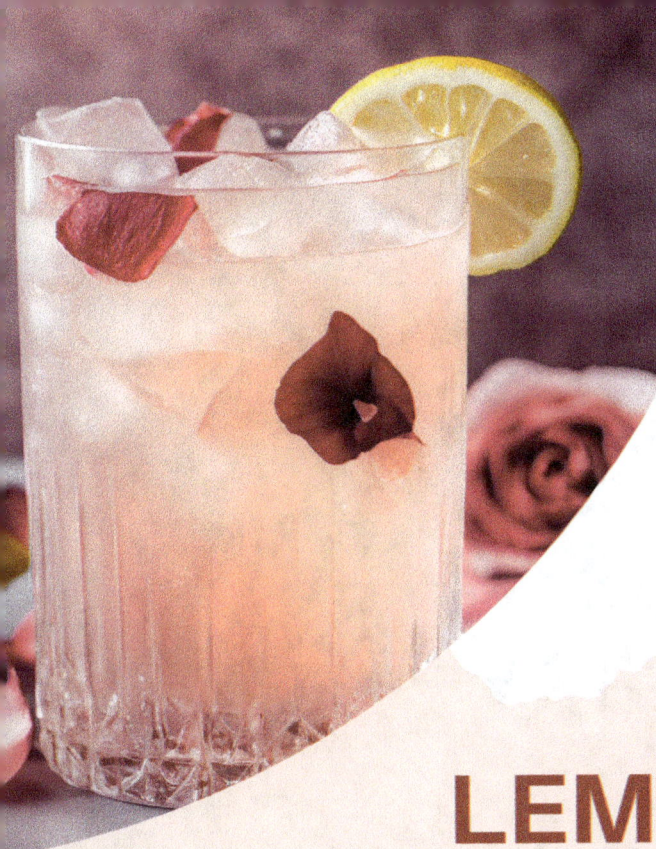

*Pure romance in a glass! The delicate sweetness of lemonade infused with the intoxicating fragrance of rose petals. It's as elegant as a garden party and as enchanting as a first kiss. This exquisite mocktail is perfect for weddings, bridal showers, or any celebration where you want to add a touch of floral magic.*

# ROSE PETAL LEMONADE

## Ingredients

- 1 cup fresh lemon juice (from about 6-8 lemons
- 1/2 cup Rose Syrup (Page 74)
- 3 cups sparkling water
- Ice cubes
- Fresh rose petals (edible) and lemon slices for garnish

## Procedure

1. In a pitcher, combine the fresh lemon juice and rose syrup. Stir well.
2. Add the sparkling water and stir gently.
3. Fill four glasses with ice and pour the mocktail mixture into the glasses.
4. Garnish each glass with fresh lemon slices and rose petals before serving.

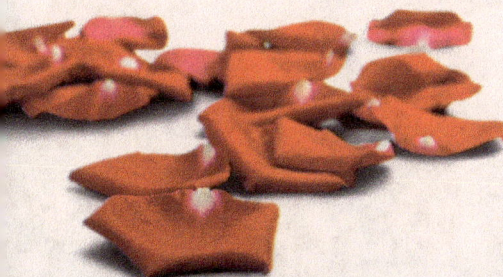

**4**
SERVING SIZE

**10** mins.
SERVING TIME

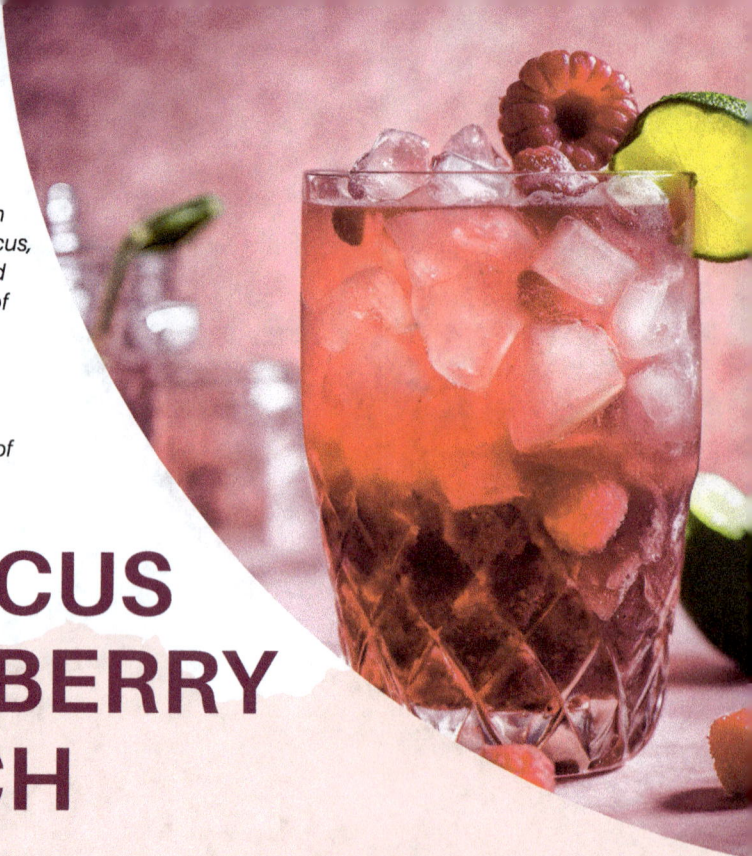

*The tart sweetness of raspberries dancing with the exotic allure of hibiscus, creating a refreshing and enchanting symphony of flavors. The perfect centerpiece for bridal showers, holiday gatherings, or elegant soirées, adding a touch of floral magic and vibrant color to any occasion.*

# HIBISCUS RASPBERRY PUNCH

## Ingredients

- 2 cups hibiscus tea (brewed and cooled from 2 tablespoons dried hibiscus flowers)
- 1 cup fresh raspberry puree (from about 1 cup of raspberries, pureed and strained
- 1/2 cup fresh lime juice (from about 4 limes)
- 3 cups soda water
- Ice cubes
- Fresh raspberries and lime wedges for garnish

## Procedure

1. In a pitcher, combine the hibiscus tea, raspberry puree and lime juice. Stir well.
2. Add the soda water and stir gently.
3. Fill four glasses with ice and pour the mocktail mixture into the glasses.
4. Garnish each glass with fresh raspberries and lime wedges before serving

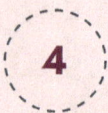

**4**

**SERVING SIZE**

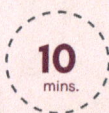

**10** mins.

**SERVING TIME**

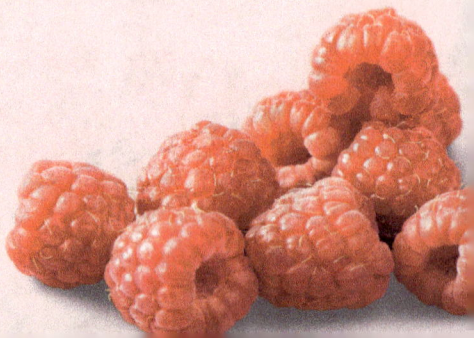

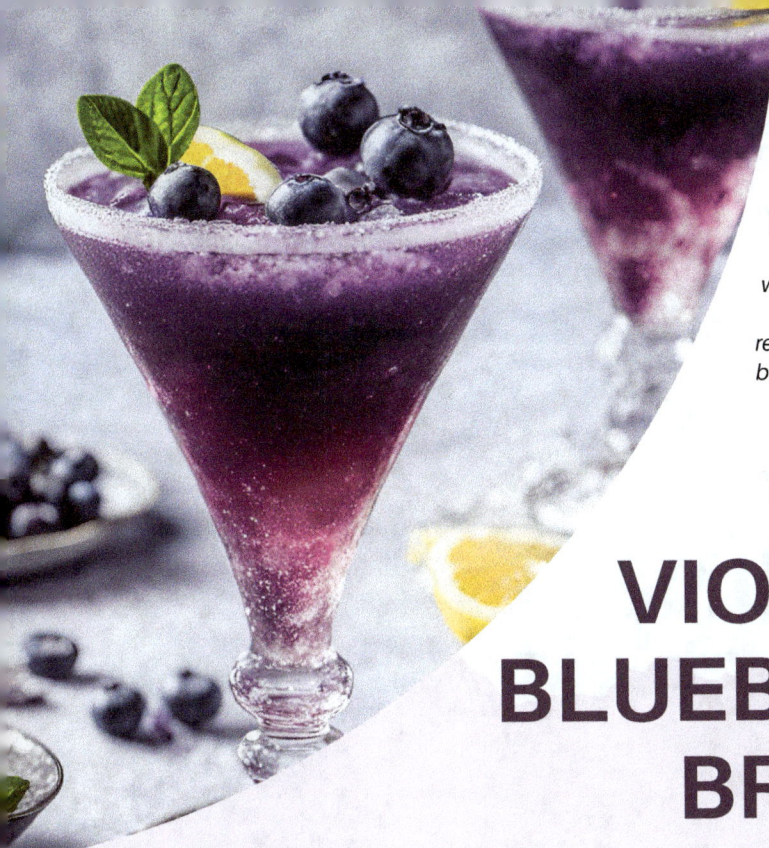

*A whisper of springtime magic! The delicate floral notes of violet mingling with the sweet juiciness of blueberries, creating a refreshing and enchanting blend of flavors, perfect for elegant soirées, garden parties, or any occasion where you want to add a touch of floral charm and whimsical delight.*

# VIOLET & BLUEBERRY BREEZE

## Ingredients

- 1 cup fresh blueberries, puree (from about 1 cup blueberries, pureed and strained)
- 1/2 cup Violet Syrup (Page 73)
- 1/2 cup fresh lemon juice
- 3 cups sparkling water
- Ice cubes
- Fresh blueberries and violet flowers (edible) for garnish

## Procedure

1. In a pitcher, combine the blueberry puree, violet syrup and lemon juice. Stir well.
2. Add the sparkling water and stir gently.
3. Fill four glasses with ice and pour the mocktail mixture into the glasses.
4. Garnish each glass with fresh blueberries and violet flowers before serving.

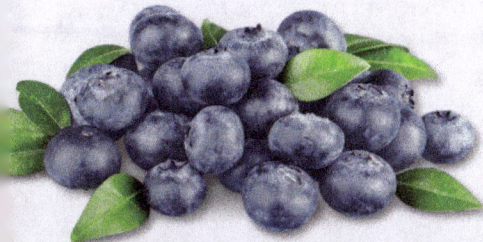

**4**

SERVING SIZE

**10** mins.

SERVING TIME

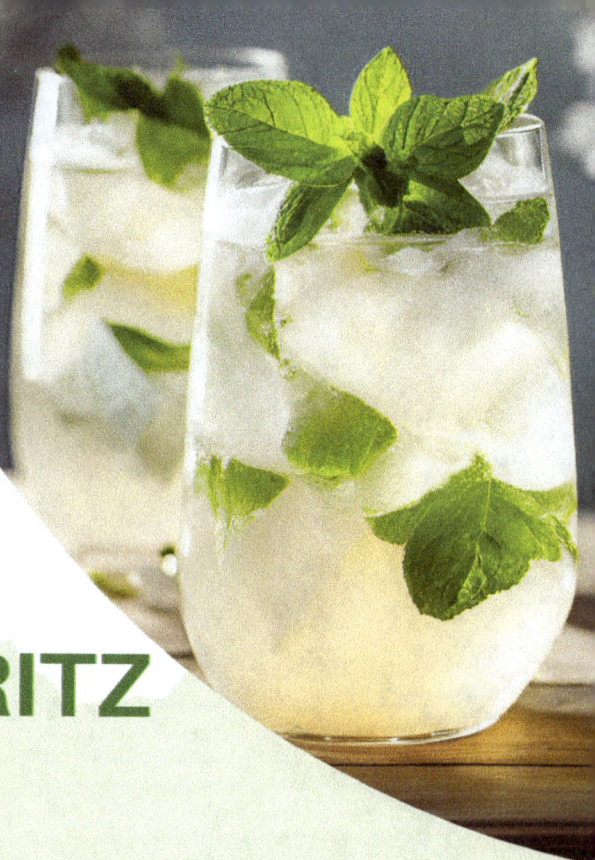

*Delightfully fragrant and refreshingly crisp, the Jasmine Pear Spritz combines the delicate floral notes of jasmine with the natural sweetness of ripe pear. A splash of sparkling water adds effervescence, creating a light, elegant mocktail that's perfect for brunches, garden parties, or a soothing evening sip. This sophisticated blend is as beautiful to look at as it is to drink.*

# JASMINE PEAR SPRITZ

## Ingredients

- 2 cups fresh pear juice (from about 4 ripe pears, pureed and strained)
- 1 cup jasmine tea (brewed and cooled from 2 jasmine tea bags)
- 3 cups soda water
- Ice cubes
- Fresh jasmine flowers (edible) and pear slices for garnish

## Procedure

1. In a pitcher, combine the pear juice and jasmine tea. Stir well.
2. Add the soda water and stir gently.
3. Fill four glasses with ice (if using) and pour the mocktail mixture into the glasses.
4. Garnish with jasmine flowers and pear slices before serving.

**4**
SERVING SIZE

**10** mins.
SERVING TIME

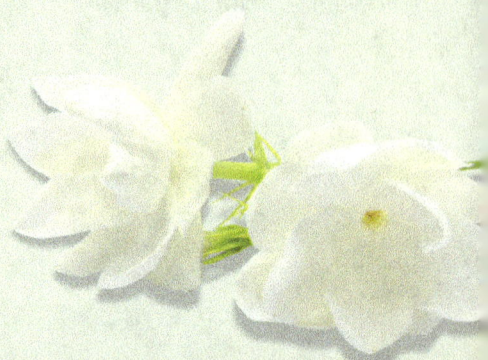

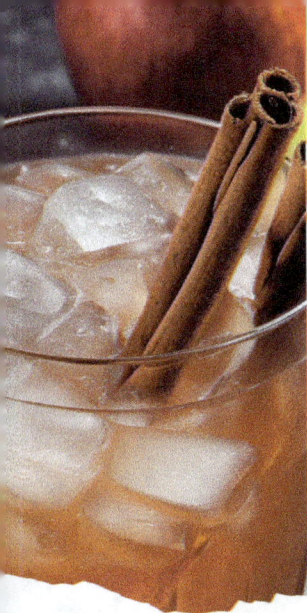

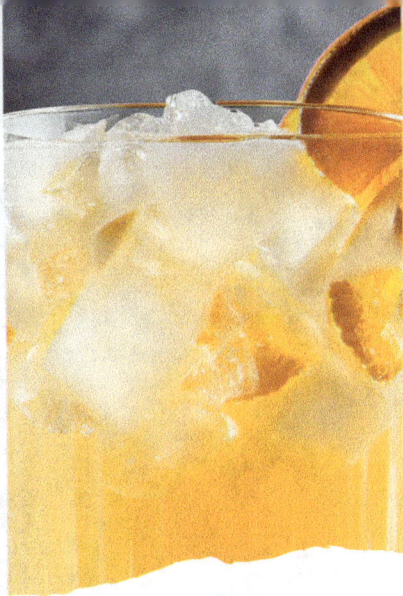

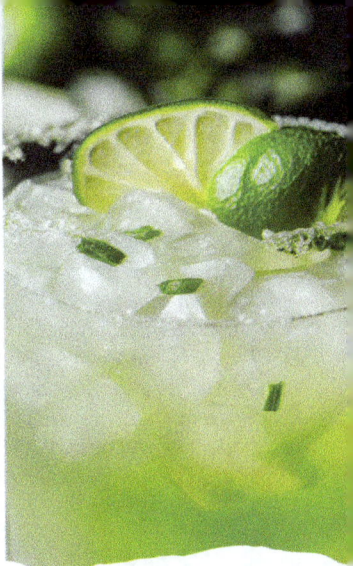

# AROMATIC INFUSIONS

These infused mocktails bring bold flavors and an aromatic twist, making them perfect for a refreshing and unique experience.

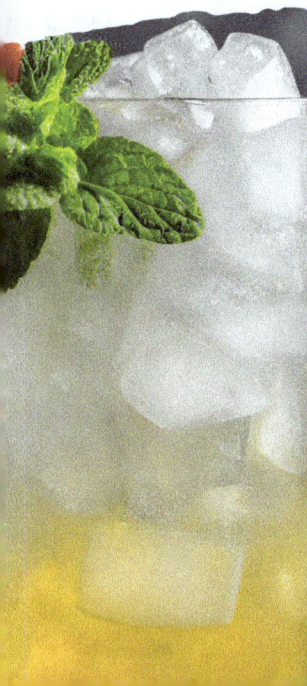

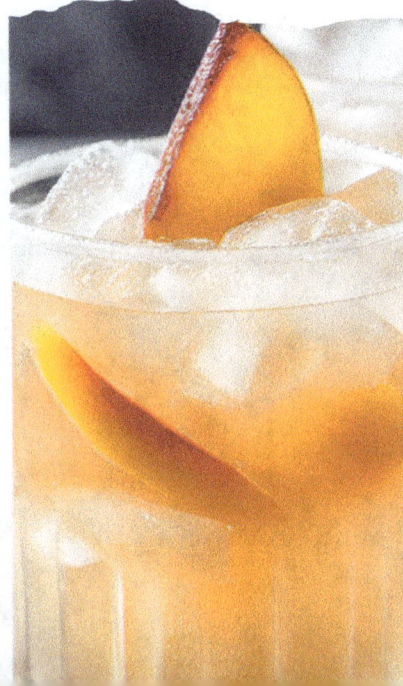

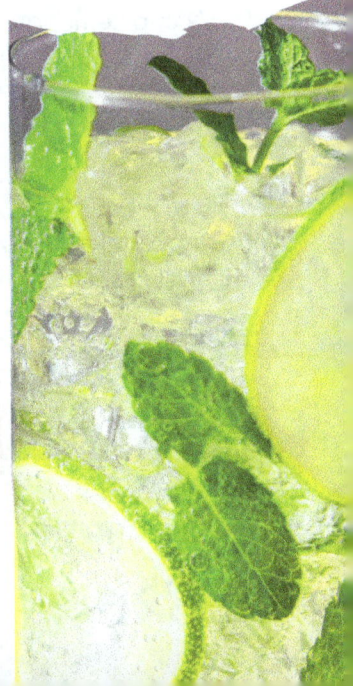

*A sip of pure serenity! The bright aroma of lemongrass intertwined with the gentle warmth of ginger, creating a harmonious blend that invigorates the senses. It's a sophisticated and refreshing mocktail, perfect for wellness retreats, spa days, or even an Asian-inspired tea party.*

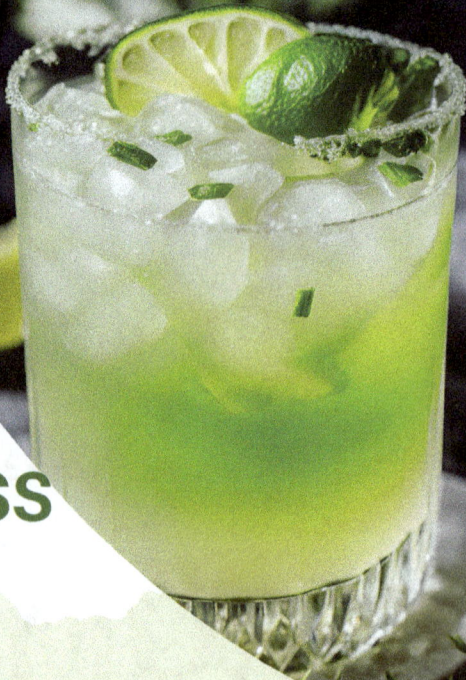

# LEMONGRASS GINGER COOLER

## Ingredients

- 2 cups fresh ginger juice (from about 4 inches of ginger root, grated and juiced)
- 1/2 cup Lemongrass Syrup (Page 73)
- 1/2 cup fresh lime juice (from about 4 limes)
- 3 cups lime soda
- Ice cubes
- Fresh lemongrass stalks and lime slices for garnish.

## Procedure

1. In a pitcher, combine the ginger juice, lemongrass syrup and lime juice. Stir well.

2. Add the lime soda and stir gently

3. Fill four glasses with ice and pour the mocktail mixture into the glasses.

4. Garnish with lemongrass stalks and lime slices before serving.

**4**

**SERVING SIZE**

**10** mins.

**SERVING TIME**

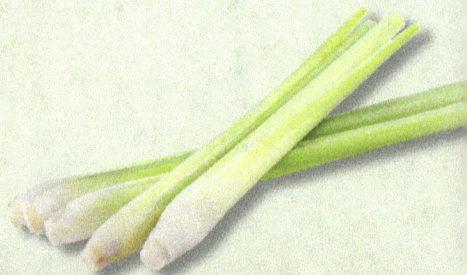

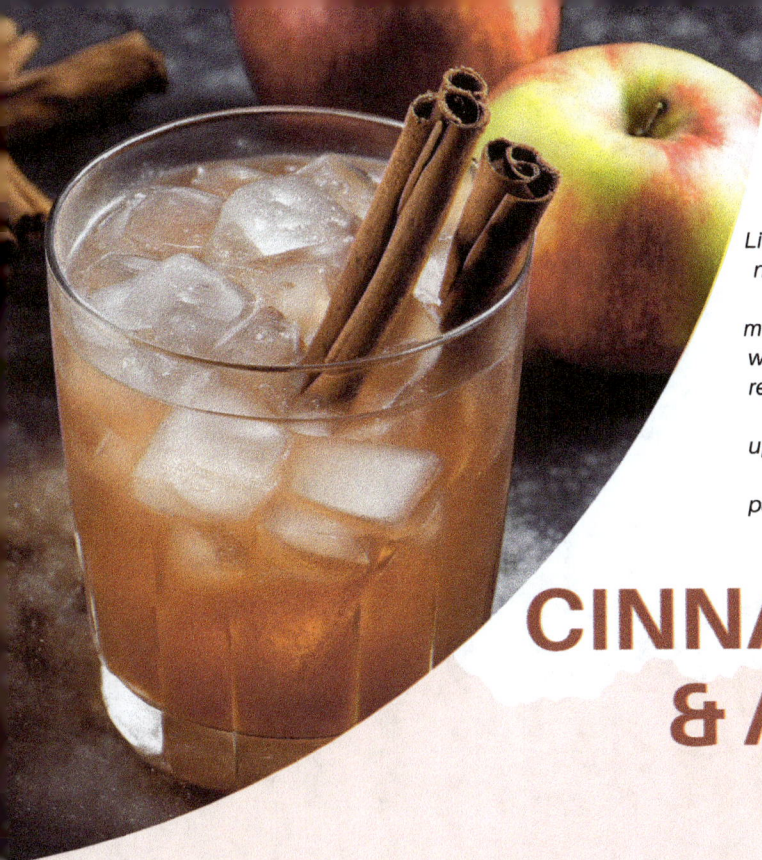

*Like a warm hug on a chilly night, the sweet and spicy flavors of apple cider mingle with the comforting warmth of cinnamon and a refreshing ginger beer fizz. The perfect drink to cozy up with by the fire, to share with friends at a holiday party, or to simply enjoy on a crisp autumn evening.*

# CINNAMON & APPLE MULE

## Ingredients

- 2 cups fresh apple juice (from about 4 apples, juiced)
- 1/2 cup Cinnamon Infusion (Page 70)
- 1 cup ginger beer (non-alcoholic)
- 3 cups soda water
- Ice cubes
- Cinnamon sticks and apple slices for garnish.

## Procedure

1. In a pitcher, combine the apple juice and cinnamon infusion. Stir well.
2. Add the ginger beer and soda water. Stir gently.
3. Fill four glasses with ice and pour the mocktail mixture into the glasses.
4. Garnish each glass with a cinnamon stick and apple slice before serving.

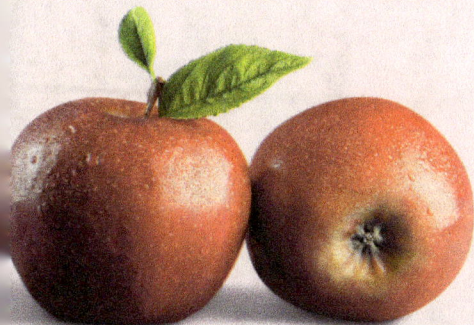

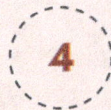

**4**

**SERVING SIZE**

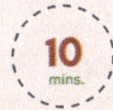

**10** mins.

**SERVING TIME**

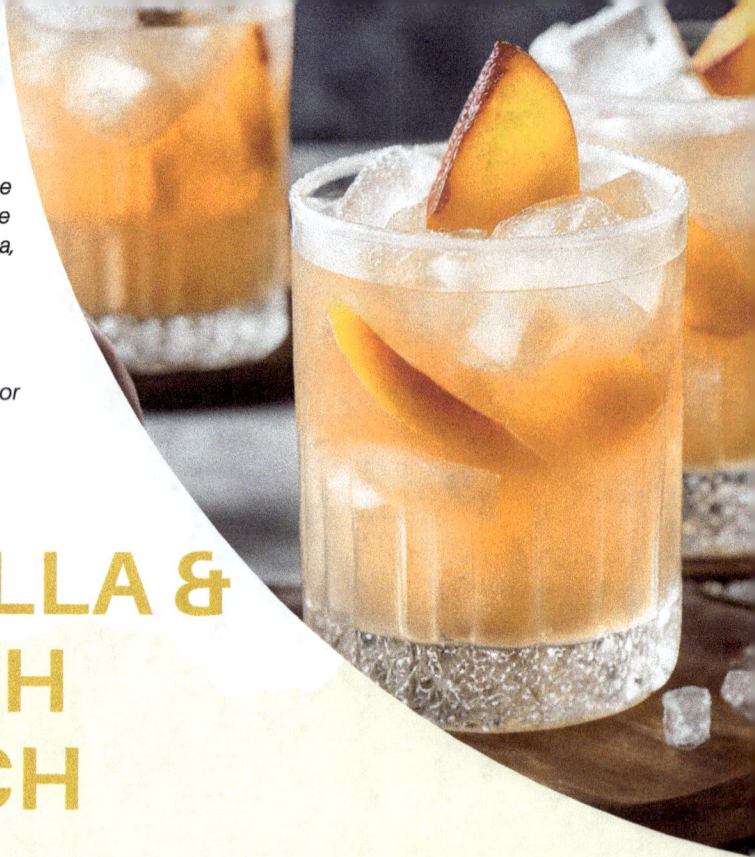

*Sweetness and charm! The luscious flavor of ripe peaches swirling with the creamy essence of vanilla, creating an elegant and refreshing harmony of flavors. A perfect centerpiece for bridal showers, baby showers, or garden parties, adding a touch of sophistication and sweetness to any celebration.*

# VANILLA & PEACH PUNCH

## Ingredients

- 2 cups fresh peach puree (from about 4 ripe peaches, pureed and strained)
- 1/2 cup Vanilla Bean Syrup (Page 76)
- 3 cups tonic water
- Ice cubes
- Fresh peach slices and vanilla beans for garnish

## Procedure

1. In a pitcher, combine the fresh peach puree and vanilla bean syrup. Stir well.
2. Add the tonic water and stir gently.
3. Fill four glasses with ice and pour the mocktail mixture into the glasses.
4. Garnish each glass with peach slices and vanilla beans before serving

**4**
SERVING SIZE

**10** mins.
SERVING TIME

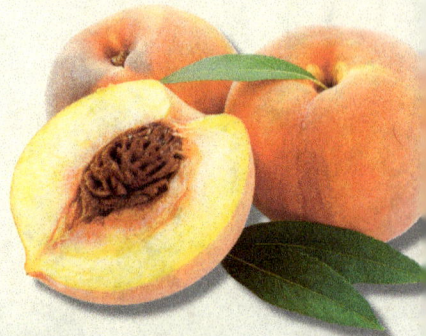

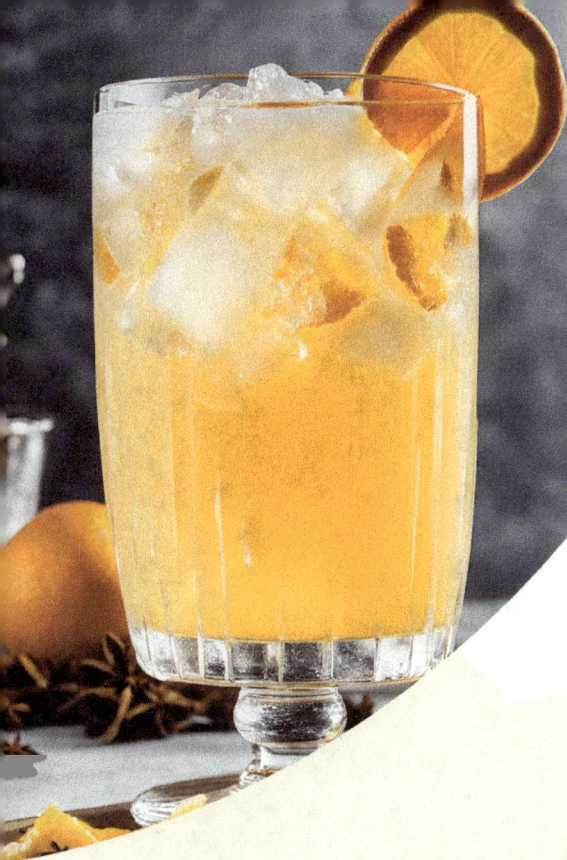

*A burst of sunshine on a crisp autumn day! The zesty brightness of orange blended with the warm embrace of cinnamon and cloves, topped with a sparkling fizz. It's festive and refreshing, perfect for holiday gatherings, cozy fireside chats, or any occasion where you want to add a touch of spice and sparkle.*

# SPICED ORANGE SPRITZ

## Ingredients

- 2 cups fresh orange juice (from about 4-5 oranges)
- 1/2 cup Spiced Clove Syrup (Page 76)
- 3 cups soda water
- Ice cubes
- Fresh orange slices and cloves for garnish.

## Procedure

1. In a pitcher, combine the fresh orange juice and spiced clove syrup. Stir well.
2. Add the soda water and stir gently.
3. Fill four glasses with ice and pour the mocktail mixture into the glasses.
4. Garnish with fresh orange slices and a few whole cloves before serving.

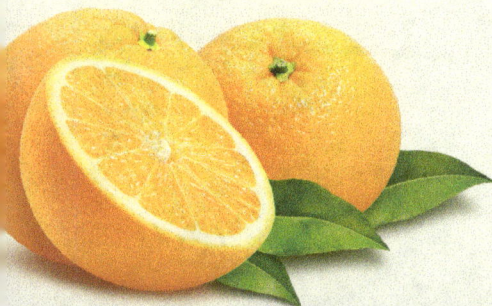

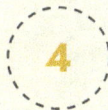

**4**

**SERVING SIZE**

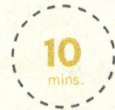

**10** mins.

**SERVING TIME**

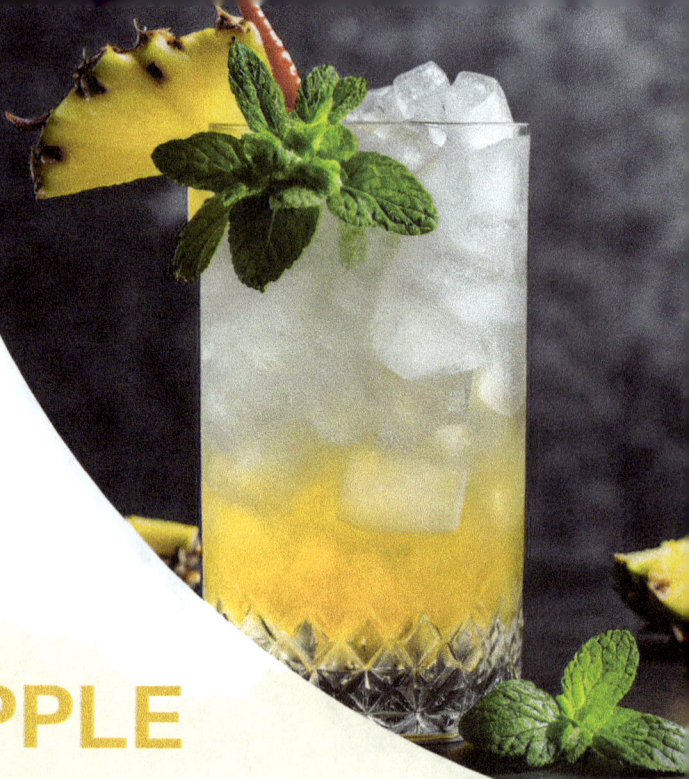

*Not for the faint of heart! The sweet juicy coolness of pineapple collides with the fiery kick of chilli peppers, blended with refreshing mint and lime. It's a daring and delicious mocktail for those who like their drinks with a bit of a bite and perfect for tropical-themed parties, summer barbecues.*

# CHILLI PINEAPPLE MOJITO

## Ingredients

- 2 cups fresh pineapple juice (from about 1 smaill pineapple)
- 1/2 cup Chilli-infused Syrup (Page 75)
- 1/2 cup fresh lime juice (from about 4 limes)
- 3 cups soda water
- Ice cubes
- Fresh mint leaves and chilli slices for garnish

## Procedure

1. In a pitcher, combine the pineapple juice, chilli-infused syrup and lime juice. Stir well.
2. Add the soda water and stir gently.
3. Fill four glasses with ice and pour the mocktail mixture into the glasses.
4. Garnish each glass with fresh mint leaves and a slice of chilli before serving.

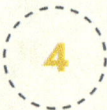

**4**

**SERVING SIZE**

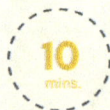

**10** mins.

**SERVING TIME**

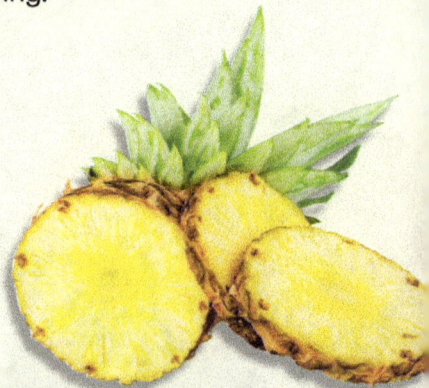

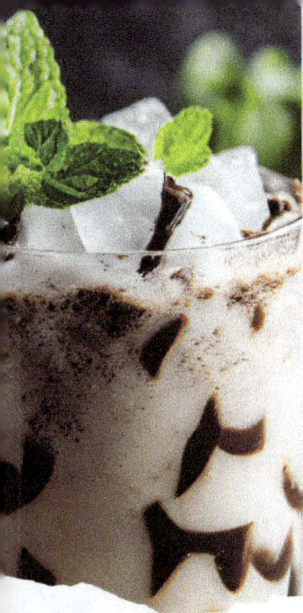

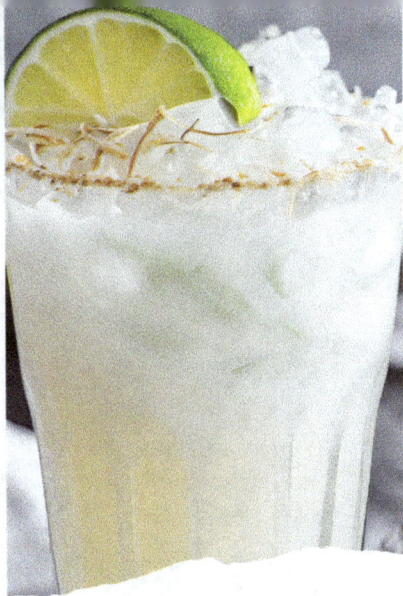

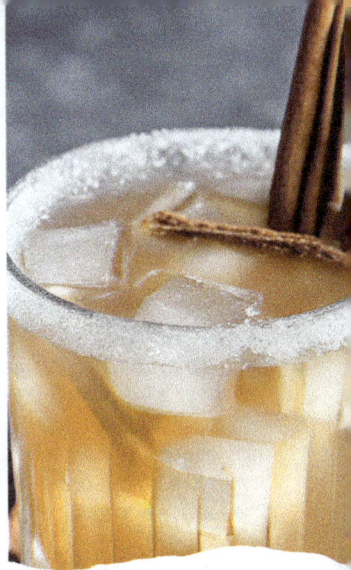

# JUST DESSERTS

*These dessert-inspired mocktails provide a sweet, indulgent treat perfect for any occasion.*

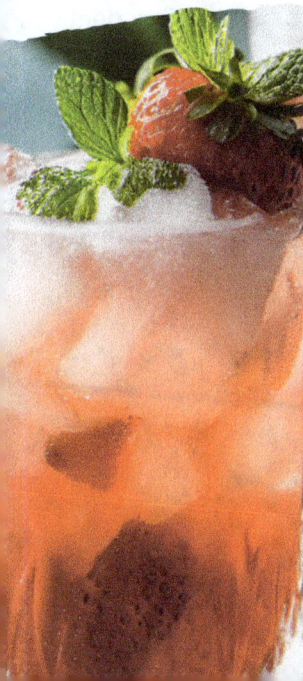

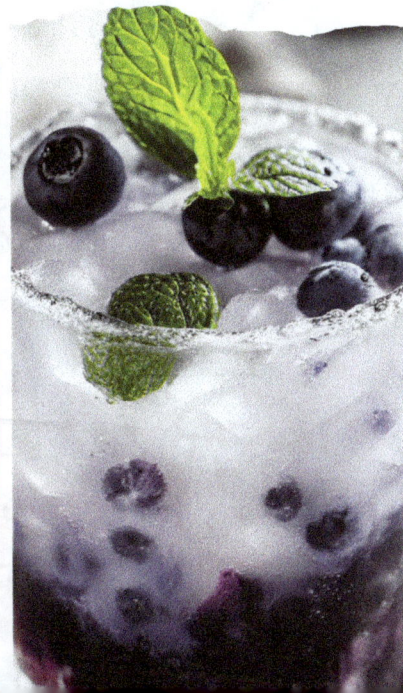

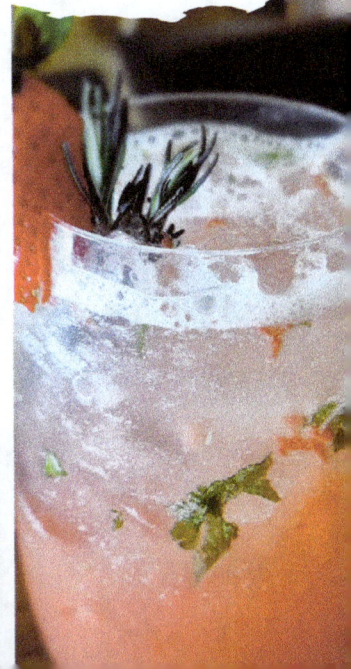

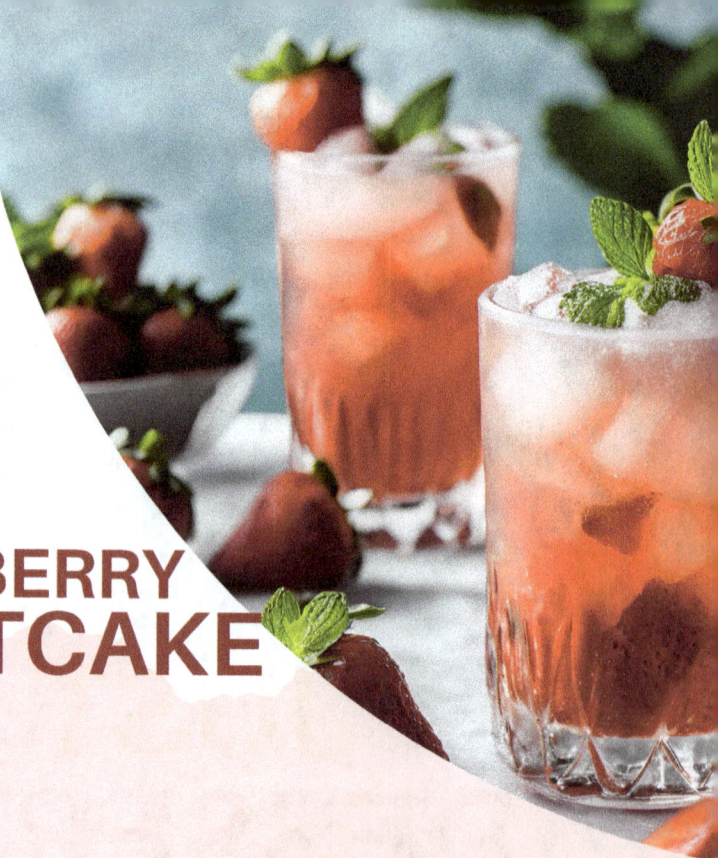

*A bubbly celebration in a glass! The sweet juiciness of strawberries and the creamy richness of vanilla, topped with a delightful fizz. A playful and refreshing mocktail, perfect for baby showers, bridal showers, or any occasion where you want to add a touch of sweetness and sparkle.*

# STRAWBERRY SHORTCAKE FIZZ

## Ingredients

- 1 cup fresh strawberry puree (from about 1 cup of strawberries, pureed and strained)
- 1/2 cup Vanilla Bean Syrup (Page 76)
- 3 cups club soda
- Ice cubes
- Fresh strawberries and mint leaves for garnish

## Procedure

1. In a pitcher, combine the strawberry puree and vanilla syrup. Stir well.
2. Add the club soda and stir gently.
3. Fill four glasses with ice and pour the mocktail mixture into the glasses.
4. Garnish with fresh strawberries and mint leaves before serving.

**4**

SERVING SIZE

**10** mins.

SERVING TIME

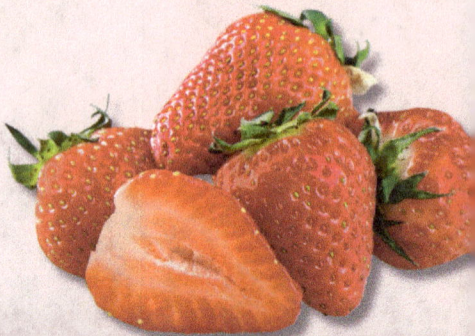

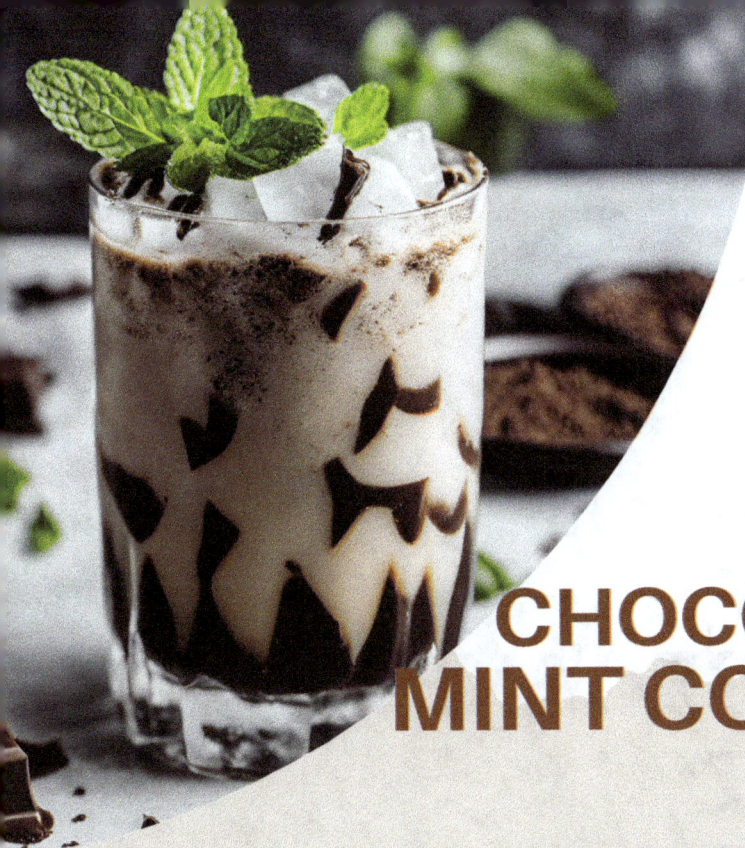

# CHOCOLATE MINT COOLER

## Ingredients

- 2 cups almond milk (or any milk of your choice)
- 1/2 cup Chocolate Syrup (Page 75)
- 1/2 cup fresh mint leaves
- Ice cubes
- Fresh mint leaves and chocolate shavings for garnish

## Procedure

1. In a pitcher, combine the almond milk and chocolate syrup. Stir well.
2. Muddle the fresh mint leaves to release the aroma, then add them to the pitcher.
3. Fill four glasses with ice and pour the mocktail mixture into the glasses.
4. Garnish with fresh mint leaves and chocolate shavings before serving

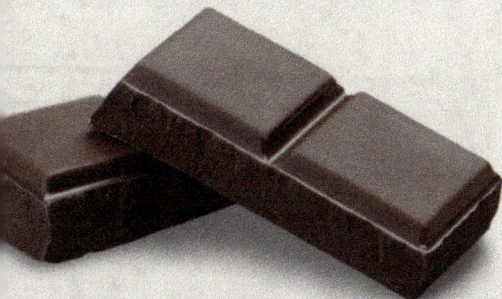

**4**
SERVING SIZE

**10** mins.
SERVING TIME

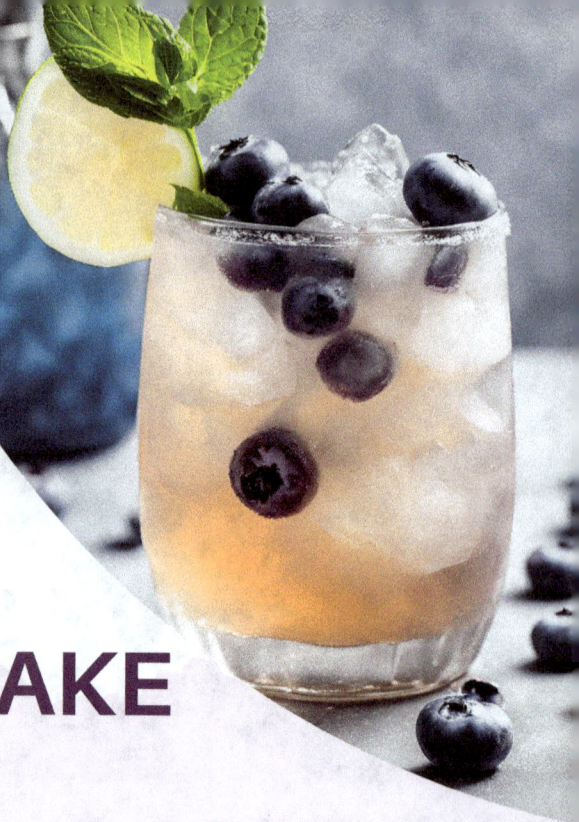

*The sweet, tangy burst of fresh berries mingled with creamy cheesecake richness, all topped with a sparkling fizz. This playful and refreshing mocktail is perfect for baby showers, garden parties, or any occasion where you want to add a touch of sweetness and indulgence.*

# BERRY CHEESECAKE SPRITZ

## Ingredients

- 1 cup fresh blueberries, pureed and strained.
- 1/2 cup cream soda
- 1/2 cup Vanilla Bean Syrup (Page 76)
- 3 cups soda water
- Ice cubes
- Fresh blueberries and a spring of mint for garnish

## Procedure

1. In a pitcher, combine the blueberry puree, cream soda and vanilla syrup. Stir well.

2. Add the soda water and stir gently.

3. Fill four glasses with ice and pour the mocktail mixture into the glasses.

4. Garnish with fresh blueberries and a sprig of mint before serving

**4**
**SERVING SIZE**

**10** mins.
**SERVING TIME**

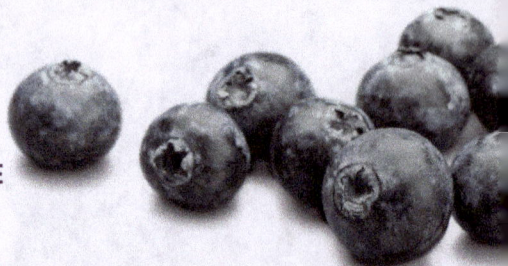

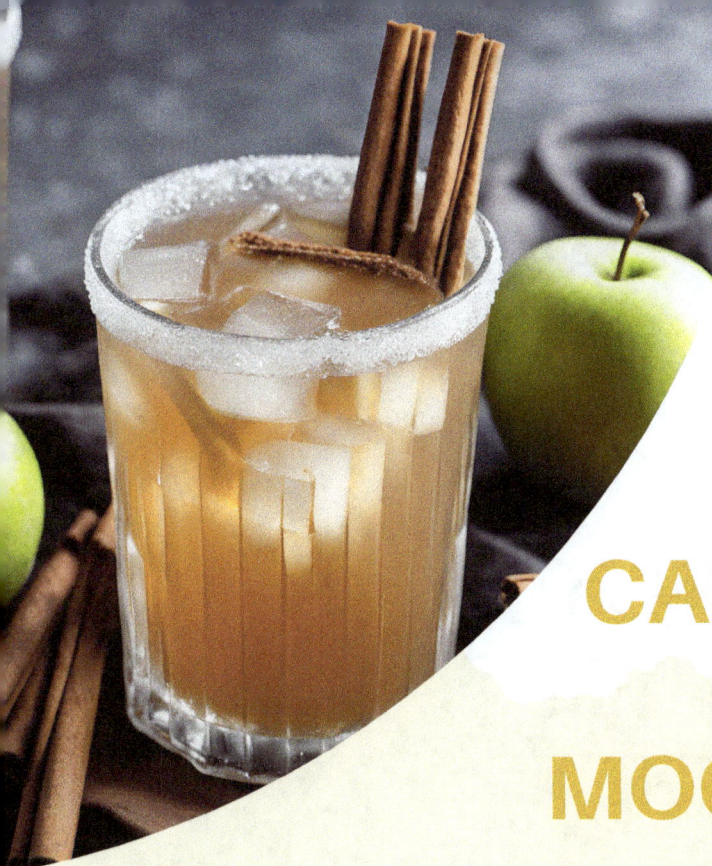

*Like a warm hug in a glass! The sweet and comforting flavors of caramel apples, with a hint of cinnamon and spice, blended into a delicious and refreshing drink. It will bring a touch of autumn magic to any fall gathering, Halloween party, or Thanksgiving dinner.*

# CARAMEL APPLE MOCKTAIL

## Ingredients

- 2 cups fresh apple juice (from about 4 apples)
- 1/2 cup Caramel Syrup (Page 77)
- 1/2 teaspoon ground cinnamon
- 3 cups soda water
- Ice cubes
- Apple slices and a cinnamon stick for garnish

## Procedure

1. In a pitcher, combine the apple juice, caramel syrup and ground cinnamon. Stir well.
2. Add the soda water and stir gently.
3. Fill four glasses with ice and pour the mocktail mixture into the glasses.
4. Garnish with apple slices and a cinnamon stick before serving.

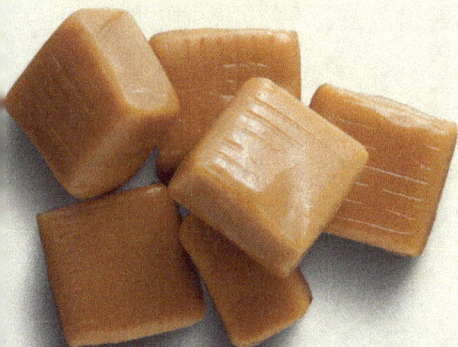

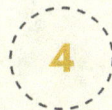

**4**

**SERVING SIZE**

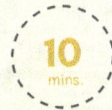

**10** mins.

**SERVING TIME**

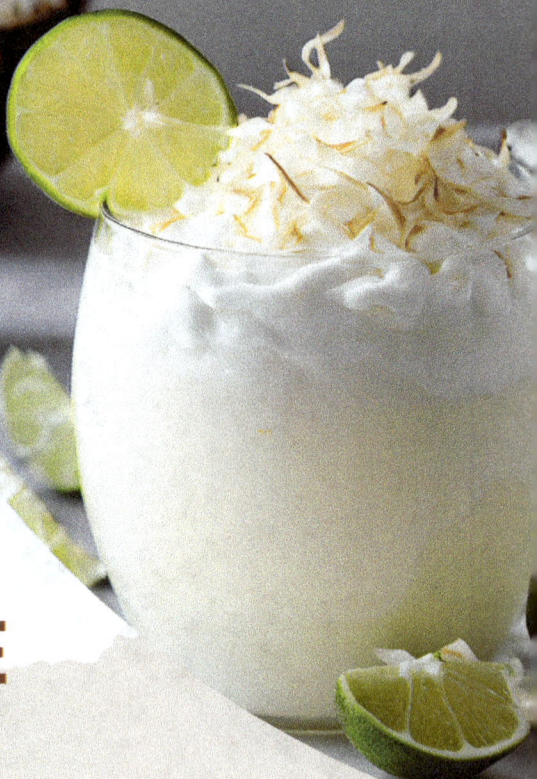

*Escape to a tropical paradise with the Coconut Cream Pie Cooler. Like a vacation in a glass, it blends luscious flavors of coconut, tangy lime, and sweet vanilla. It's the perfect way to cool down on a hot day, transport yourself to a beachside cabana, or simply indulge in a moment of pure bliss.*

# COCONUT CREAM PIE COOLER

## Ingredients

- 2 cups coconut milk (full-fat for creaminess)
- 1/2 cup lime juice (from about 4 limes)
- 1/2 cup Vanilla Bean Syrup (Page 76)
- Ice cubes
- Toasted coconut flakes and lime slices for garnish

## Procedure

1. In a pitcher, combine the coconut milk, lime juice, and vanilla syrup. Stir well.

2. Fill four glasses with ice (if using) and pour the mocktail mixture into the glasses.

3. Garnish with toasted coconut flakes and lime slices before serving.

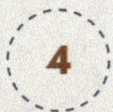

**4**

**SERVING SIZE**

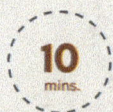

**10** mins.

**SERVING TIME**

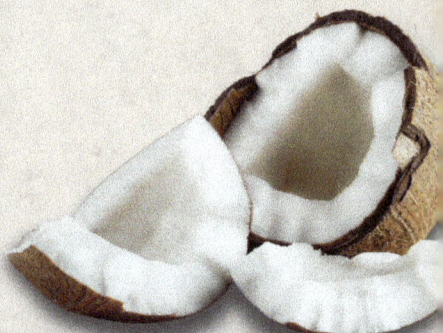

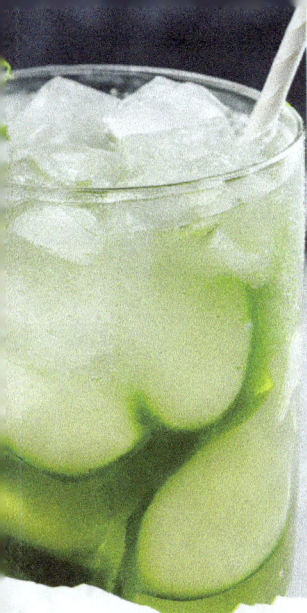

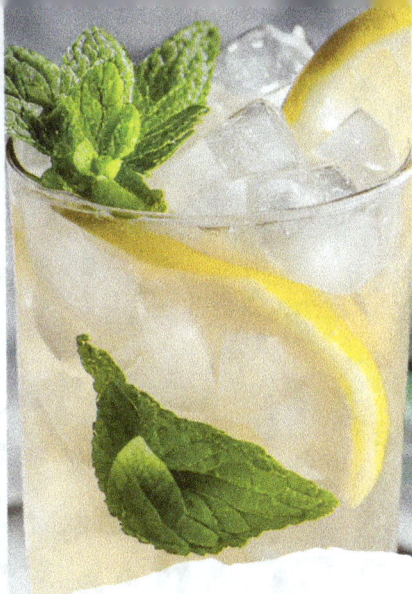

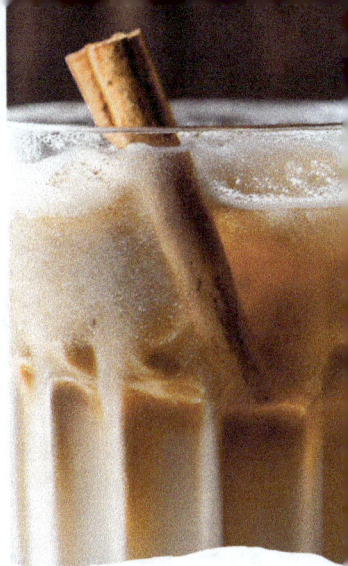

# TEA-BASED
## COCKTAILS

*These tea-based mocktails offer a refreshing and sophisticated experience, combining classic tea flavors with refreshing twists.*

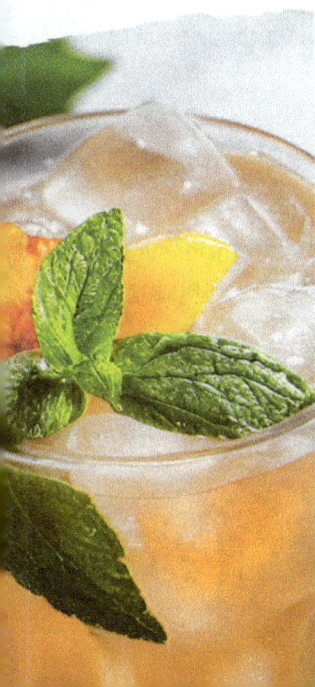

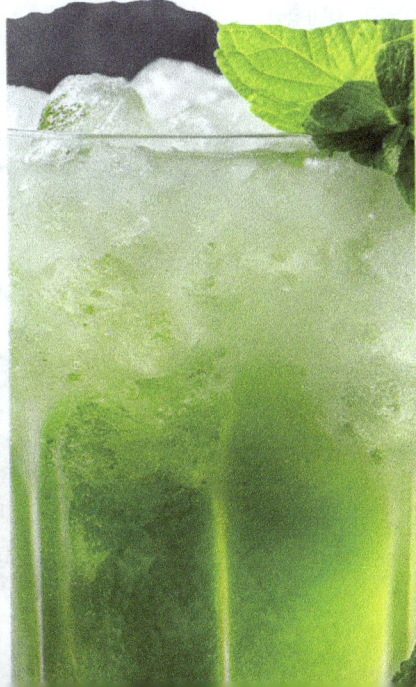

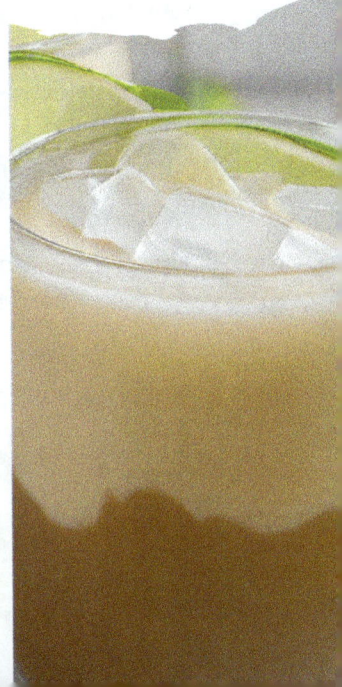

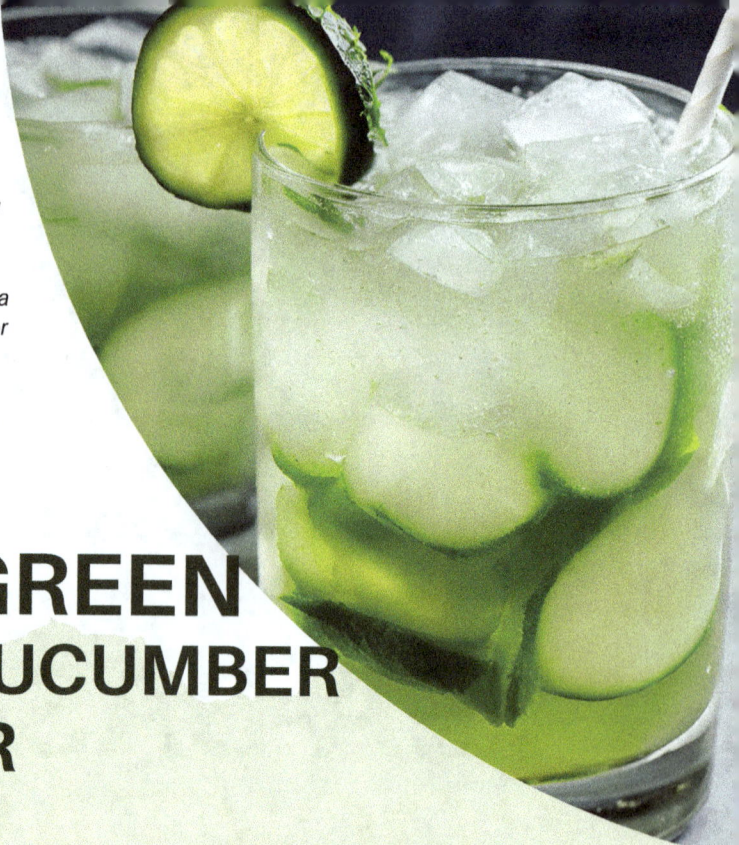

*Pure refreshment in a glass! Crisp, clean green tea combined with cool, refreshing cucumber. Like a revitalizing spa treatment for your taste buds, perfect for unwinding after a yoga session, enjoying a relaxing spa day, or simply cooling down on a hot summer afternoon.*

# ICED GREEN
# TEA & CUCUMBER
# COOLER

## Ingredients

- 2 cups green tea (brewed and cooled from 2 green tea bags)
- 1 cup fresh cucumber juice (from about 1 large cucumber, pureed and strained)
- 1/2 cup fresh lime juice (from about 4 limes)
- 3 cups soda water
- Ice cubes
- Cucumber slices and lime wedges for garnish.

## Procedure

1. In a pitcher, combine the cooled green tea, cucumber juice and lime juice. Stir well.

2. Add the soda water and stir gently.

3. Fill four glasses with ice and pour the mocktail mixture into the glasses.

4. Garnish with cucumber slices and lime wedges before serving.

**4**

**SERVING SIZE**

**10** mins.

**SERVING TIME**

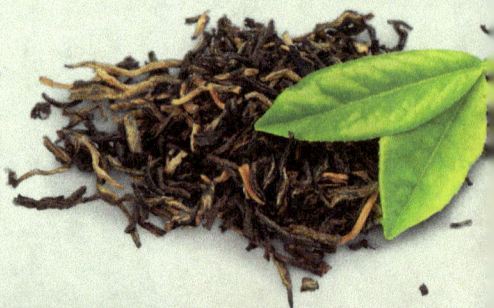

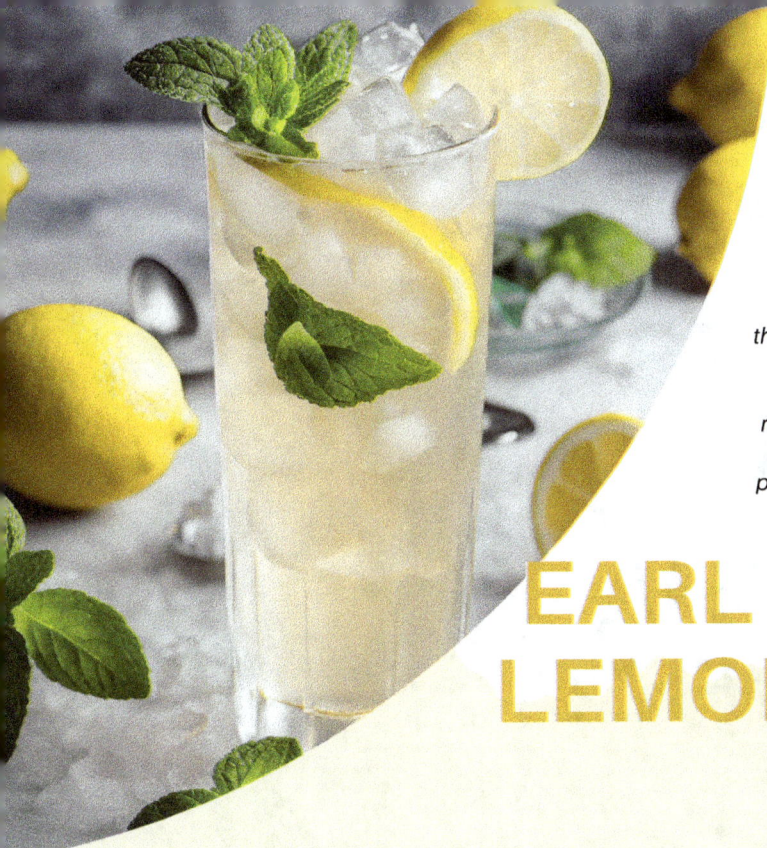

*A refined twist on a beloved classic! The bright, citrusy tang of lemonade infused with the delicate floral notes of Earl Grey tea, creates, a sophisticated and refreshing mocktail that's perfect for afternoon tea parties, bridal showers, or any elegant gathering.*

# EARL GREY LEMONADE

## Ingredients

- 2 cups brewed and cooled Earl Grey tea (from 2 tea bags)
- 1/2 cup fresh lemon juice (from about 4 lemons)
- 1/2 cup Lemon Syrup (Page 66)
- 3 cups soda water
- Ice cubes
- Lemon slices and fresh mint leaves for garnish.

## Procedure

1. In a pitcher, combine the cooled Earl Grey tea, lemon juice and lemon syrup. Stir well.
2. Add the soda water and stir gently.
3. Fill four glasses with ice and pour the mocktail mixture into the glasses.
4. Garnish with lemon slices and fresh mint leaves before serving.

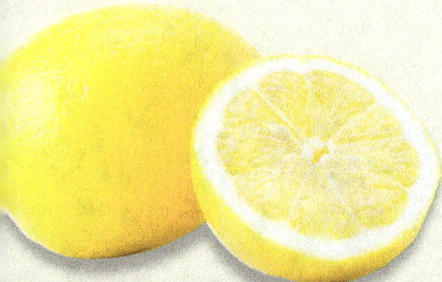

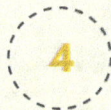

**4**

**SERVING SIZE**

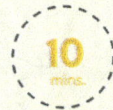

**10** mins.

**SERVING TIME**

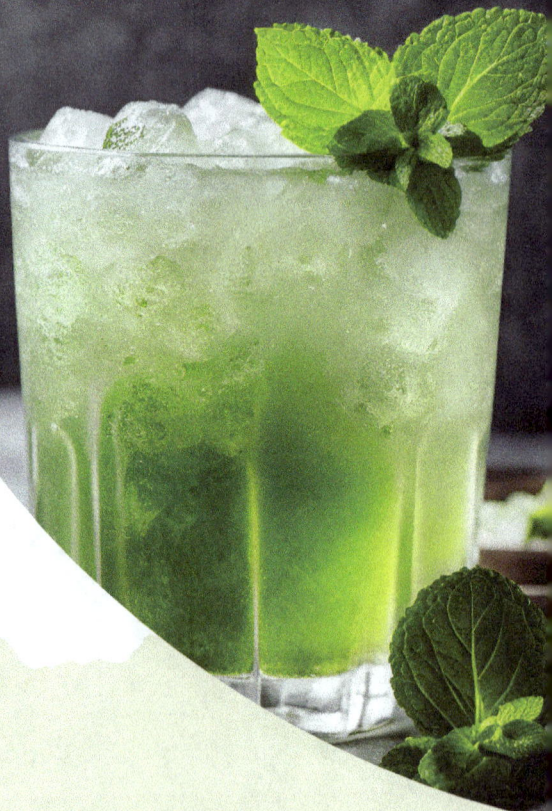

*A vibrant burst of energy and refreshment combining the earthy goodness of matcha with the invigorating coolness of mint, topped with a sparkling fizz. It's a revitalizing mocktail that's perfect for wellness retreats, yoga classes, or trendy brunches.*

# MATCHA MINT FIZZ

## Ingredients

- 2 cups water
- 2 teaspoons matcha powder
- 1/2 cup Mint Syrup (Page 66)
- 3 cups sparkling water
- Ice cubes
- Fresh mint leaves for garnish

## Procedure

1. In a pitcher, whisk the matcha powder into the water until fully dissolved.
2. Add the mint syrup and stir well.
3. Add the sparkling water and stir gently.
4. Fill four glasses with ice and pour the mocktail mixture into the glasses.
5. Garnish with fresh mint leaves before serving

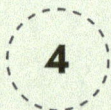

**4**

**SERVING SIZE**

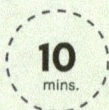

**10** mins.

**SERVING TIME**

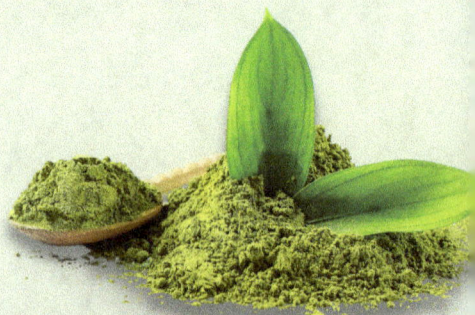

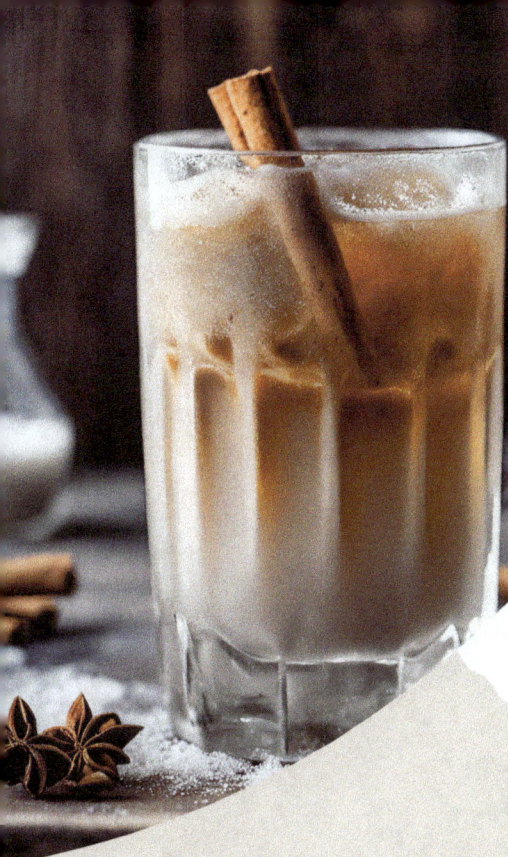

*The comforting warm spices of chai tea – cinnamon, cardamom, ginger – mingled with refreshing milky coolness, creating a delightful harmony of flavors. It's the perfect drink to cozy up with on a chilly evening, share with friends at a holiday party, or simply enjoy while curled up with a good book.*

# CHAI SPICE COOLER

## Ingredients

- 2 cups brewed and cooled chai tea (from 2 chai tea bags)
- 1/2 cup Cinnamon Syrup (Page 67)
- 1 cup almond milk (or any milk of your choice
- Ice cubes
- Ground cinnamon for garnish

## Procedure

1. In a pitcher, combine the cooled chai tea, cinnamon syrup and almond milk. Stir well.

2. Fill four glasses with ice and pour the mocktail mixture into the glasses.

3. Garnish each glass with a sprinkle of ground cinnamon before serving.

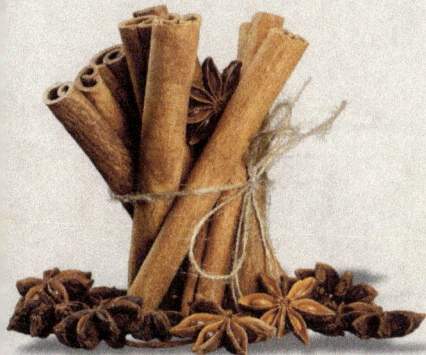

**4**

**SERVING SIZE**

**10** mins.

**SERVING TIME**

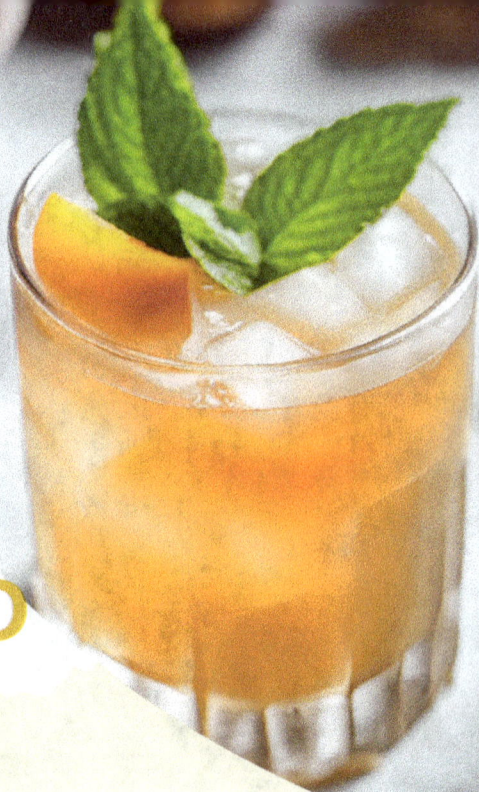

*A taste of summer in a glass! The sweet juiciness of peaches mingled with the refreshing iced tea, with a sparkling fizz. A delightful and easy-going mocktail that's perfect for summer picnics, backyard barbecues, or lazy brunches.*

# PEACH ICED TEA SPRITZ

## Ingredients

- 2 cups brewed and cooled peach tea (from 2 peach tea bags)
- 1 cup fresh peach puree (from about 2 ripe peaches, pureed and strained)
- 1/2 cup Vanilla Bean Syrup (Page 76)
- 3 cups soda water
- Ice cubes
- Fresh peach slices and mint leaves for garnish

## Procedure

1. In a pitcher, combine the cooled peach tea, peach puree and vanilla syrup. Stir well.
2. Add the soda water and stir gently.
3. Fill four glasses with ice and pour the mocktail mixture into the glasses.
4. Garnish with fresh peach slices and mint leaves before serving.

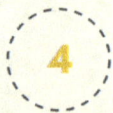

**4**

SERVING SIZE

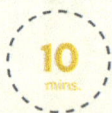

**10** mins.

SERVING TIME

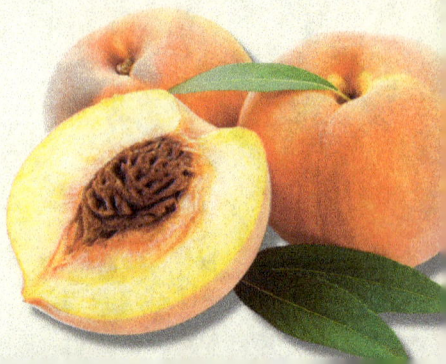

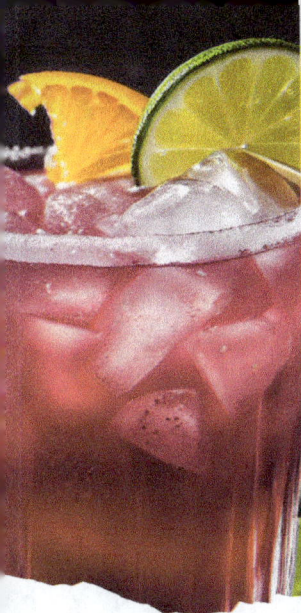

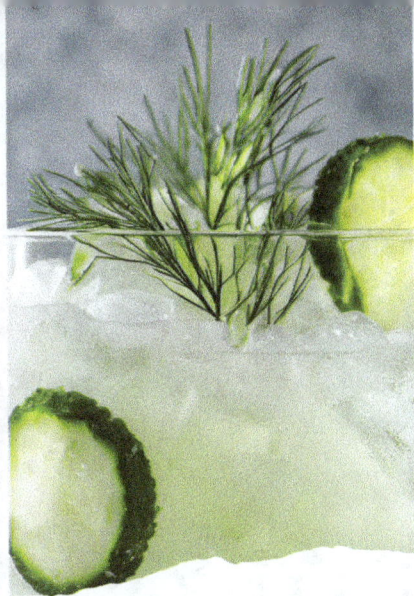

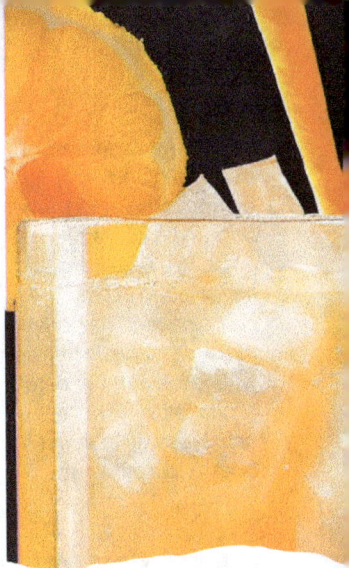

# WITH A TWIST

These unique and experimental mocktails provide a refreshing and innovative experience, combining bold flavors and fresh ingredients.

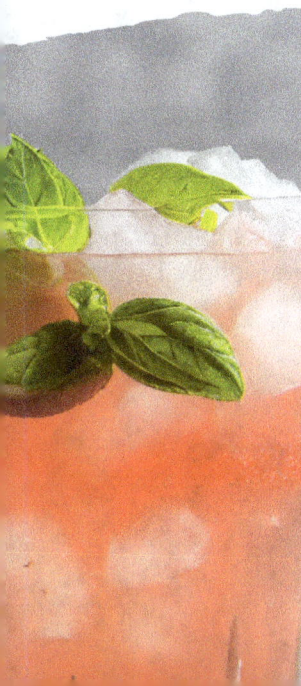

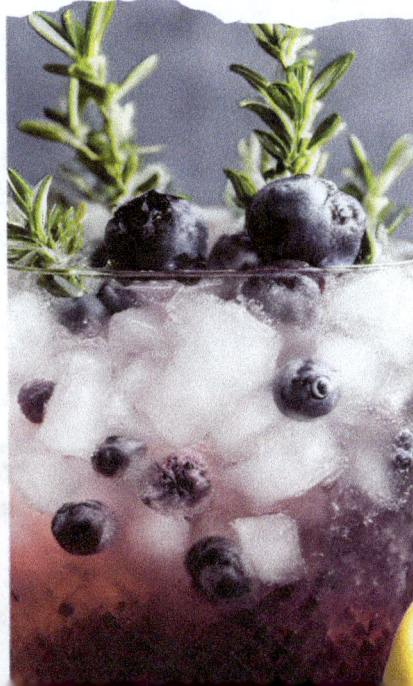

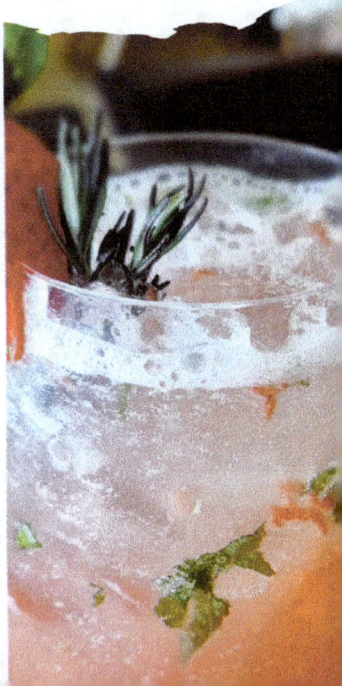

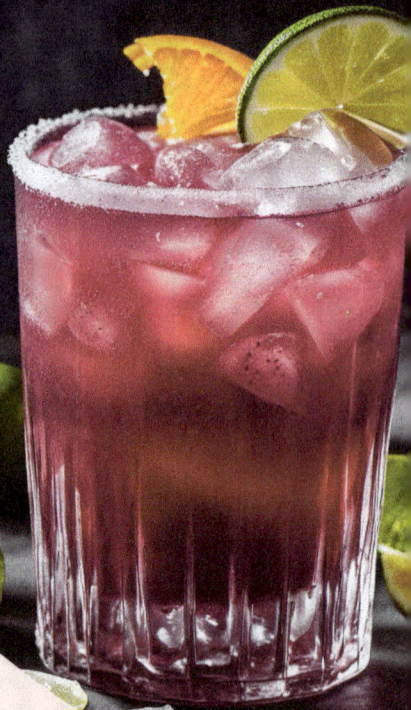

*The earthy sweetness of beetroot blending harmoniously with the zesty brightness of orange, creating a refreshing and invigorating flavor combination. The perfect mocktail for health retreats, wellness events, or detox brunches, offering a delicious way to nourish your body and awaken your senses.*

# BEETROOT & ORANGE ZEST COOLER

## Ingredients

- 1 cup fresh beet juice (from about 2 medium beets)
- 1/2 cup Orange Syrup (Page 67)
- 1/2 cup fresh lime juice (from about 4 limes)
- 3 cups soda water
- Ice cubes
- Fresh orange slices and lime wedges for garnish.

## Procedure

1. In a pitcher, combine the beet juice, orange syrup and lime juice. Stir well.

2. Add the soda water and stir gently.

3. Fill four glasses with ice and pour the mocktail mixture into the glasses.

4. Garnish each glass with orange slices and lime wedges before serving.

**4**
SERVING SIZE

**10** mins.
SERVING TIME

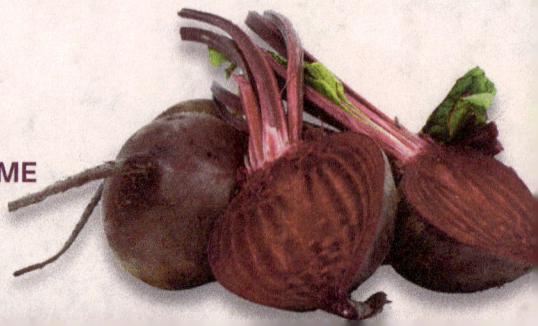

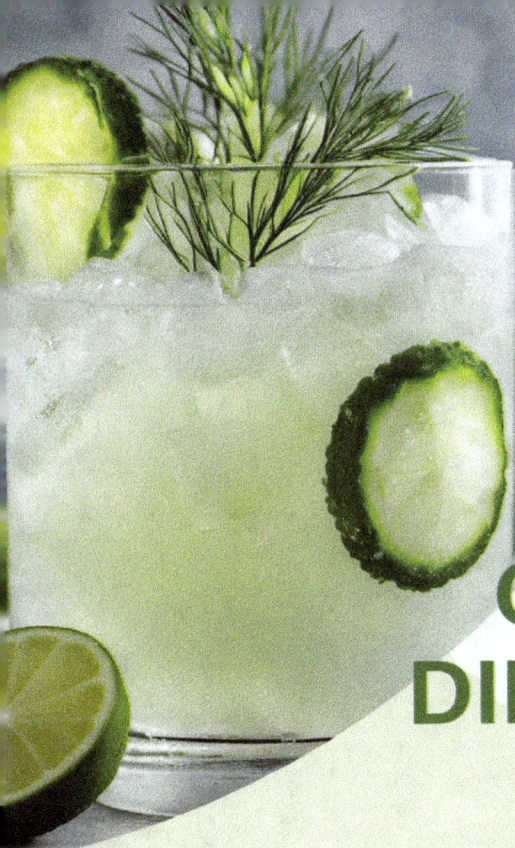

*The epitome of understated elegance! The crisp coolness of cucumber with the fresh herbaceous notes of dill, creating a sophisticated flavor profile. It's a truly refined mocktail, perfect for stylish dinner parties, cocktail hours, or garden soirées under the stars.*

# CUCUMBER DILL MARTINI

## Ingredients

- 1 cup fresh cucumber juice (from about 2 large cucumbers, pureed and strained.
- 1/2 cup Dill Infusion (Page 77)
- 1/4 cup fresh lime juice (from about 2 limes
- 3 cups soda water
- Ice cubes
- Fresh cucumber slices and dill sprigs for garnish

## Procedure

1. In a pitcher, combine the cucumber juice, dill infusion and lime juice. Stir well.
2. Add the soda water and stir gently.
3. Fill four glasses with ice and pour the mocktail mixture into the glasses.
4. Garnish each glass with cucumber slices and dill sprigs before serving.

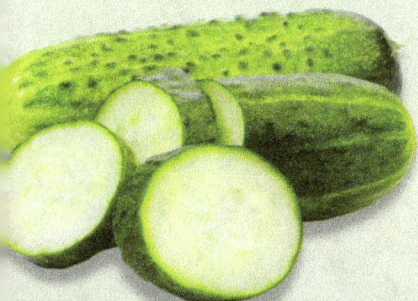

**4**
SERVING SIZE

**10** mins.
SERVING TIME

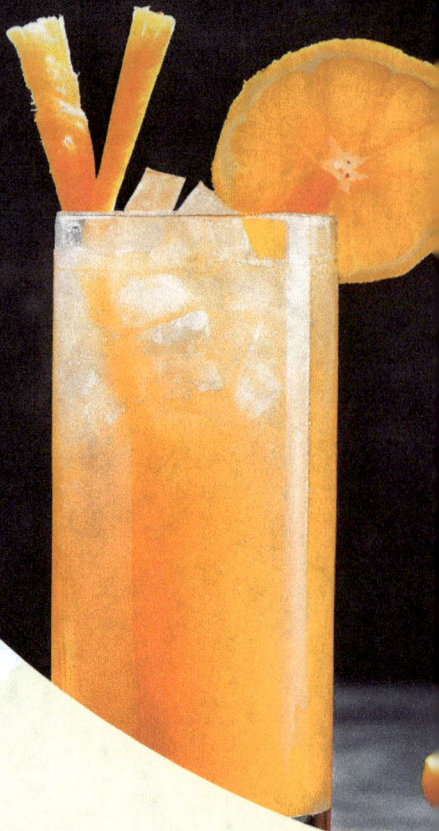

*A vibrant burst of health and flavor with carrot sweetness and the invigorating warmth of ginger, creating a revitalizing elixir that's as delicious as it is good for you. The perfect mocktail for health retreats, autumn brunches, or any time you want to boost your immunity and tantalize your taste buds.*

# CARROT GINGER PUNCH

## Ingredients

- 2 cups fresh carrot juice (from about 6 medium carrots)
- 1/2 cup Ginger Syrup (Page 68)
- 1/2 cup fresh orange juice (from about 2 oranges)
- 3 cups soda water
- Ice cubes
- Fresh carrot sticks and orange slices for garnish

## Procedure

1. In a pitcher, combine the carrot juice, ginger syrup and orange juice. Stir well.
2. Add the soda water and stir gently.
3. Fill four glasses with ice and pour the mocktail mixture into the glasses.
4. Garnish with carrot sticks and orange slices before serving.

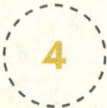

**4**

**SERVING SIZE**

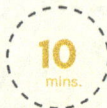

**10** mins.

**SERVING TIME**

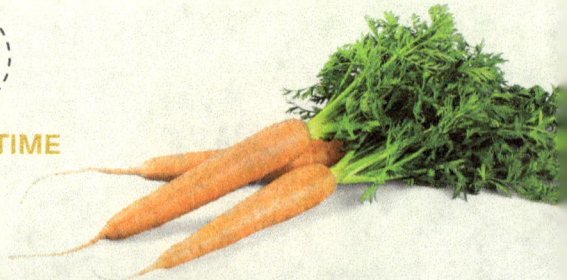

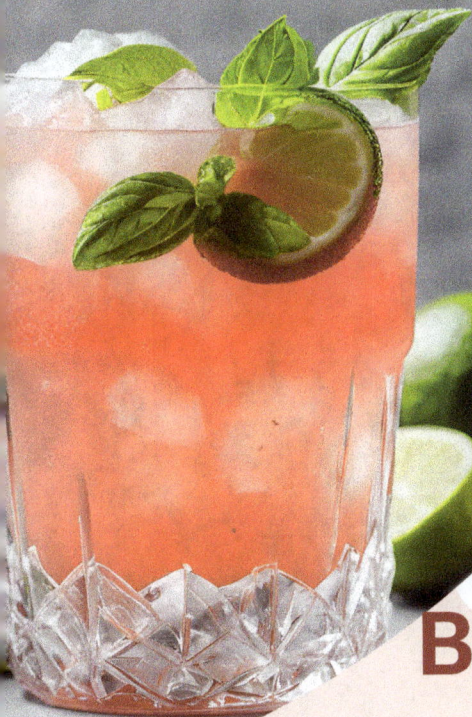

*A taste of summer in a glass! The juicy sweetness of watermelon collides with fragrant basil, creating a refreshing mocktail perfect for poolside lounging, backyard barbecues, or beach picnics. It offers a delightful way to cool down and refresh on a hot summer's day.*

# WATERMELON
# BASIL SMASH

## Ingredients

- 2 cups fresh watermelon juice (from about 1/4 of a medium watermelon, pureed and strained)
- 1/2 cup Basil Syrup (Page 68)
- 1/2 cup fresh lime juice (from about 4 limes)
- 3 cups soda water
- Ice cubes
- Fresh basil leaves and lime wedges for garnish.

## Procedure

1. In a pitcher, combine the watermelon juice, basil syrup and lime juice. Stir well.

2. Add the soda water and stir gently.

3. Fill four glasses with ice and pour the mocktail mixture into the glasses.

4. Garnish with basil leaves and lime wedges before serving.

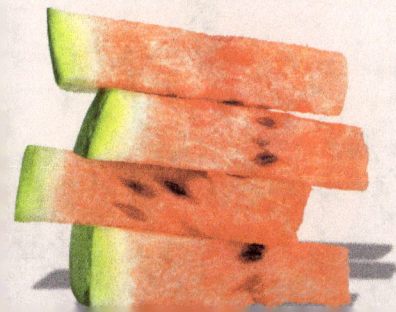

**4**
SERVING SIZE

**10** mins.
SERVING TIME

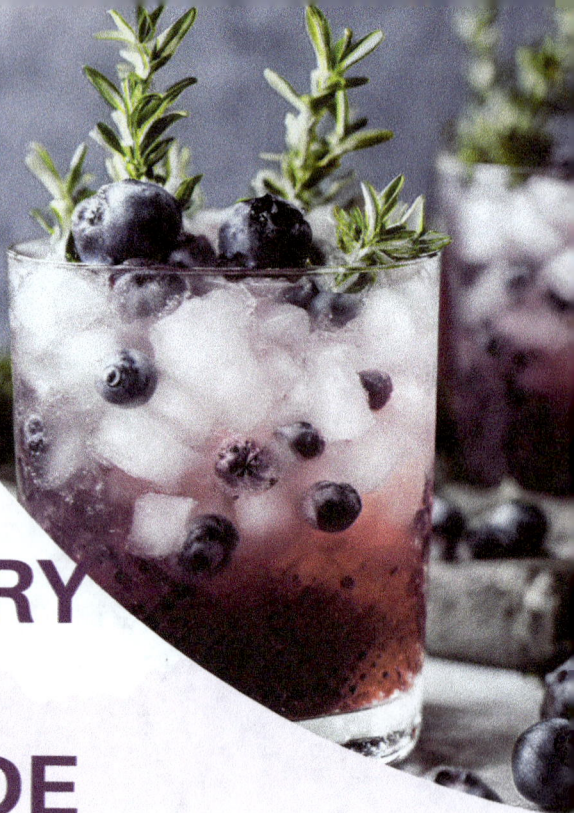

*A burst of summertime sweetness with the juicy sweetness of blueberries dancing with the zesty tang of lemonade, infused with delicate thyme. It's a refreshing and delightful mocktail perfect for baby showers, garden parties, or any occasion where you want to add a touch of floral charm and summertime bliss.*

# BLUEBERRY THYME LEMONADE

## Ingredients

- 1 cup fresh blueberry puree (from about 1 cup blueberries, pureed and strained)
- 1/2 cup Thyme Syrup (Page 72)
- 2 cups fresh lemon juice (from about 6-8 lemons)
- 3 cups soda water
- Ice cubes
- Fresh blueberries and thyme sprigs for garnish

## Procedure

1. In a pitcher, combine the blueberry puree, thyme syrup and lemon juice. Stir well.
2. Add the soda water and stir gently.
3. Fill four glasses with ice and pour the mocktail mixture into the glasses.
4. Garnish with fresh blueberries and thyme sprigs before serving.

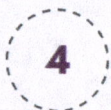

**4**

**SERVING SIZE**

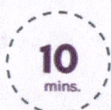

**10** mins.

**SERVING TIME**

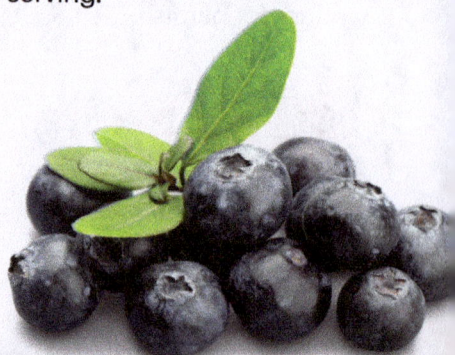

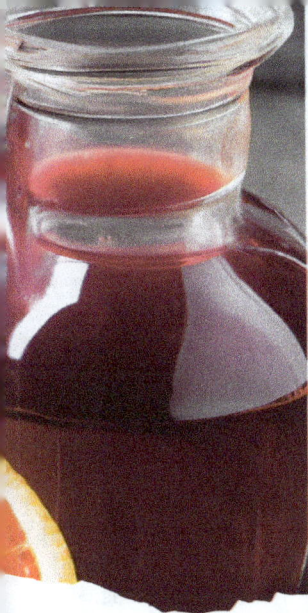

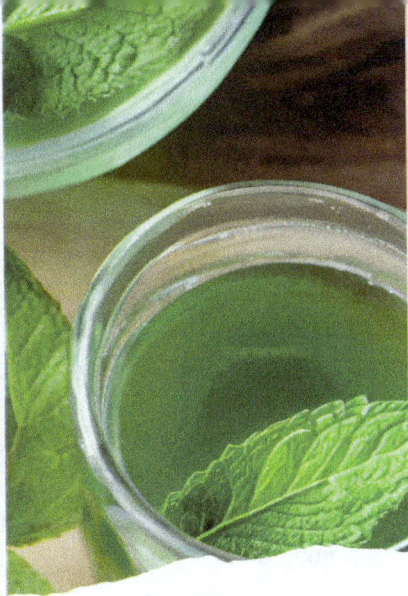

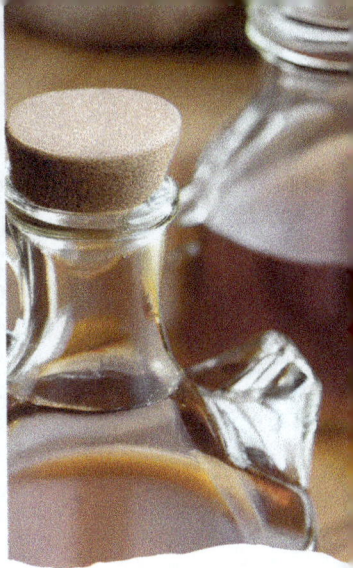

# SYRUPS, INFUSIONS AND CORDIALS

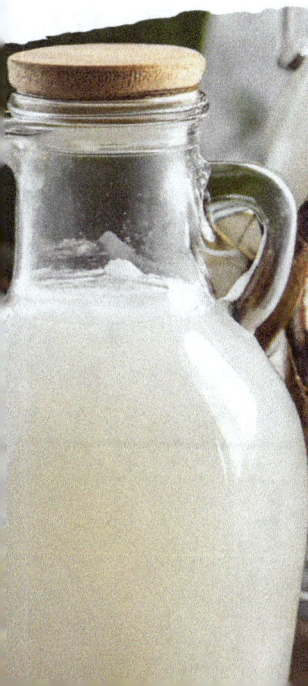

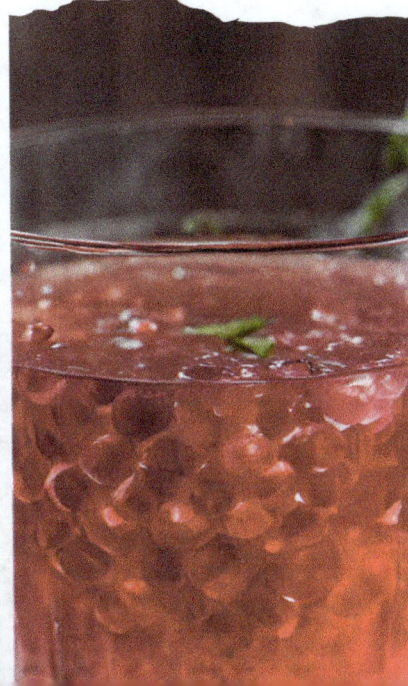

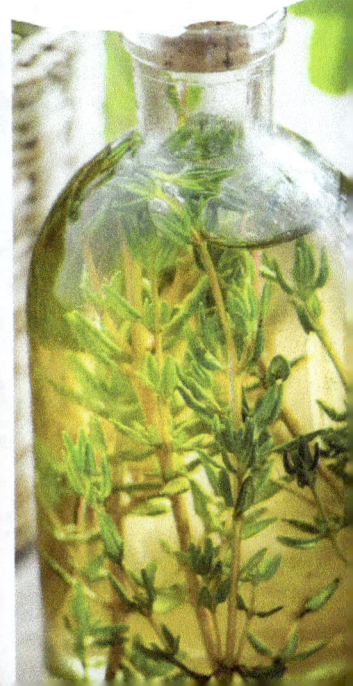

# HOMEMADE GRENADINE

## Ingredients

- 1 cup fresh pomegranate juice (from about 2 large pomegranates)
- 1 cup granulated sugar

## Procedure

1. In a saucepan, combine the pomegranate juice and sugar. Bring to a boil, then reduce the heat and simmer for 5 minutes.
2. Remove from heat and let it cool before using. Store in a sterilized bottle in the refrigerator for up to 2 weeks.

# LIME CORDIAL

## Ingredients

- 1 cup fresh lime juice (from about 8-10 limes)
- 1 cup water
- 1 cup granulated sugar

## Procedure

1. In a saucepan, combine lime juice, water, and sugar. Bring to a boil, then reduce the heat and simmer for 5 minutes until the sugar is dissolved.
2. Let the cordial cool before using.

# MINT SYRUP

## Ingredients

- 1 cup water
- 1 cup granulated sugar
- 1 cup fresh mint leaves

## Procedure

1. In a saucepan, combine water, sugar, and mint leaves. Bring to a boil, then reduce the heat and simmer for 5 minutes.
2. Remove from heat and let the syrup steep for 15 minutes.
3. Strain out the mint leaves and let the syrup cool before using.

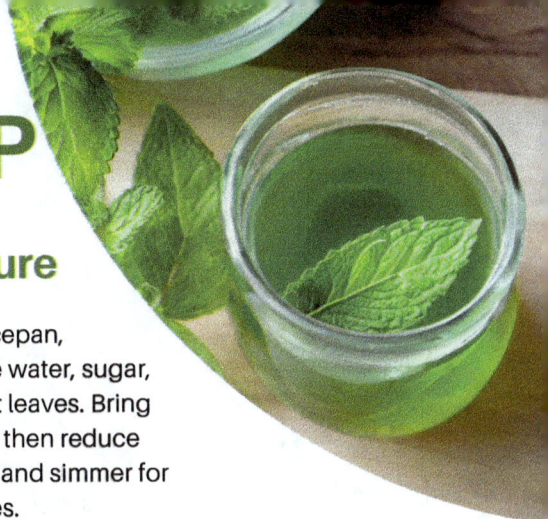

# LEMON SYRUP

## Ingredients

- 1 cup water
- 1 cup granulated sugar
- Zest of 2 lemons

## Procedure

1. In a saucepan, combine water, sugar, and lemon zest. Bring to a boil, then reduce the heat and simmer for 5 minutes.
2. Remove from heat and let the syrup cool before using.

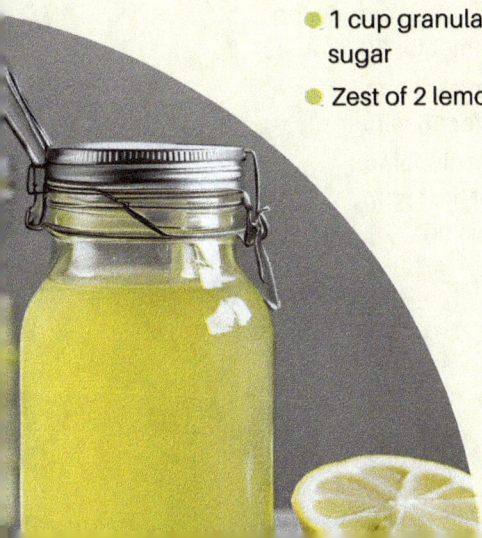

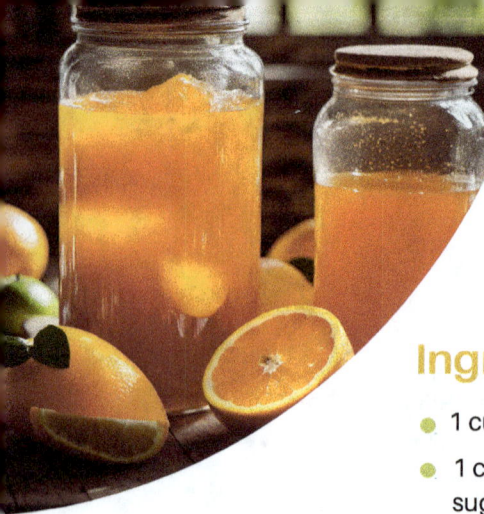

# ORANGE SYRUP

## Ingredients

- 1 cup water
- 1 cup granulated sugar
- Zest of 1 orange

## Procedure

1. In a saucepan, combine water, sugar, and orange zest. Bring to a boil, then reduce the heat and simmer for 5 minutes.
2. Remove from heat and let the syrup cool before using.

# CINNAMON SYRUP

## Ingredients

- 1 cup water
- 1 cup granulated sugar
- 3 cinnamon sticks

## Procedure

1. In a saucepan, combine water, sugar, and cinnamon sticks. Bring to a boil, then reduce the heat and simmer for 10 minutes.
2. Remove from heat and let the syrup steep for 15 minutes.
3. Strain out the cinnamon sticks and let the syrup cool before using.

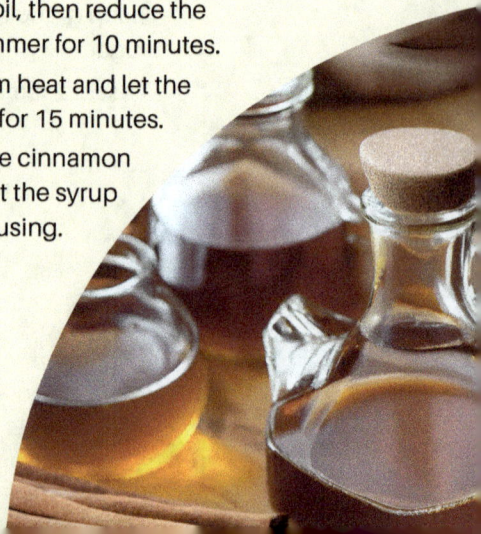

# GINGER SYRUP

## Ingredients

- 1 cup water
- 1 cup granulated sugar
- 1 cup fresh ginger root (sliced)

## Procedure

1. In a saucepan, combine water, sugar, and ginger slices. Bring to a boil, then reduce the heat and simmer for 10 minutes.
2. Remove from heat and let the syrup steep for 15 minutes.
3. Strain out the ginger slices and let the syrup cool before using.

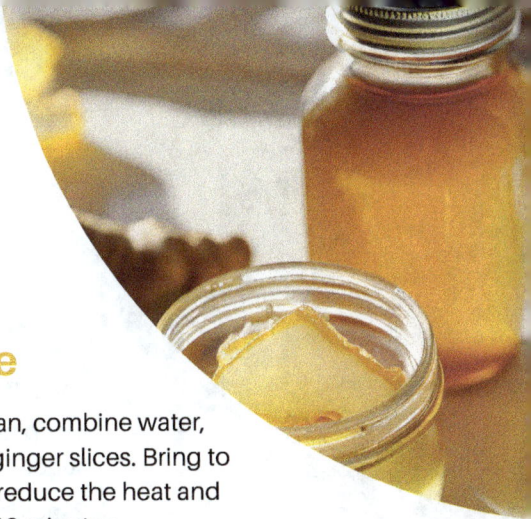

# BASIL SYRUP

## Ingredients

- 1 cup water
- 1 cup granulated sugar
- 1 cup fresh basil leaves

## Procedure

1. In a saucepan, combine water, sugar, and basil leaves. Bring to a boil, then reduce the heat and simmer for 5 minutes.
2. Remove from heat and let the syrup steep for 15 minutes.
3. Strain out the basil leaves and let the syrup cool before using.

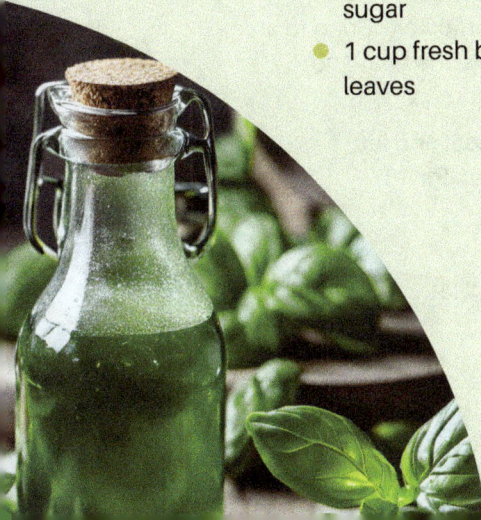

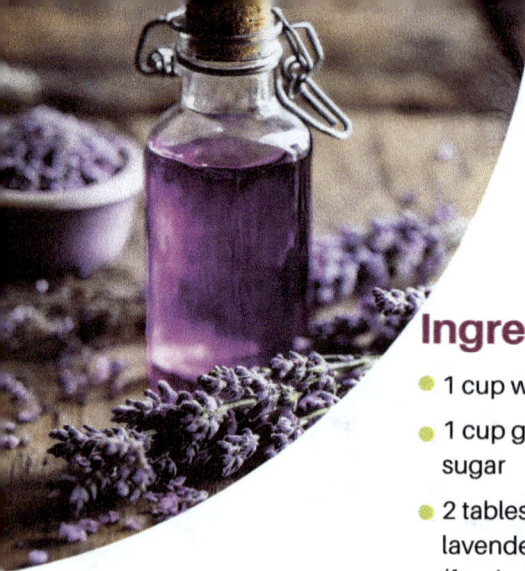

# LAVENDER SYRUP

## Ingredients

- 1 cup water
- 1 cup granulated sugar
- 2 tablespoons dried lavender flowers (food-grade)

## Procedure

1. In a saucepan, combine water, sugar, and lavender flowers. Bring to a boil, then reduce the heat and simmer for 5 minutes.
2. Remove from heat and let the syrup steep for 15 minutes.
3. Strain out the lavender flowers and let the syrup cool before using.

# ELDERFLOWER CORDIAL

## Ingredients

- 1 cup water
- 1 cup granulated sugar
- 1/2 cup dried elderflowers (or 1 cup fresh elderflowers)

## Procedure

1. In a saucepan, combine water, sugar, and elderflowers. Bring to a boil, then reduce the heat and simmer for 5 minutes.
2. Remove from heat and let the mixture steep for 15 minutes.
3. Strain out the elderflowers and let the cordial cool before using.

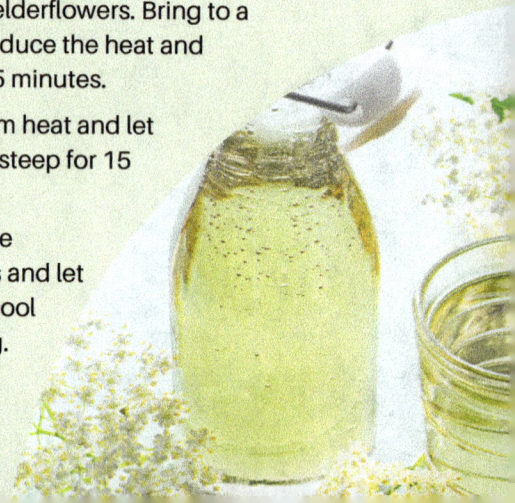

# CINNAMON INFUSION

## Ingredients

- 1 cup water
- 2 cinnamon sticks

## Procedure

1. In a saucepan, bring the water and cinnamon sticks to a boil. Reduce the heat and simmer for 5 minutes.
2. Remove from heat and let it steep for an additional 15 minutes.
3. Strain out the cinnamon sticks and let the infusion cool before using.

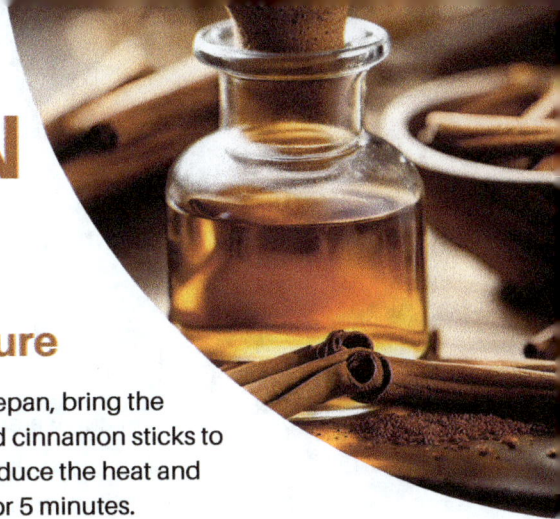

# ROSEMARY SYRUP

## Ingredients

- 1 cup water
- 1 cup granulated sugar
- 3 sprigs fresh rosemary

## Procedure

1. In a saucepan, combine water, sugar, and rosemary sprigs. Bring to a boil, then reduce the heat and simmer for 5 minutes.
2. Remove from heat and let the syrup steep for 15 minutes.
3. Strain out the rosemary sprigs and let the infusion cool before using.

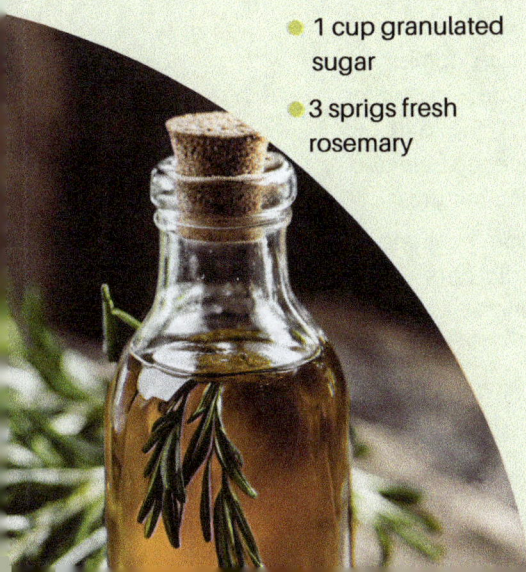

# HIBISCUS TEA

## Ingredients

- 1 cup water
- 2 tablespoons dried hibiscus flowers

## Procedure

1. Bring water to a boil, then add the dried hibiscus flowers.
2. Reduce the heat and simmer for 5 minutes. Remove from heat and let the tea steep for an additional 10 minutes.
3. Strain out the flowers and let the tea cool before using.

# POMEGRANATE CORDIAL

## Ingredients

- 1 cup water
- 1 cup granulated sugar
- 1 cup fresh pomegranate juice (from about 2 pomegranates)

## Procedure

1. In a saucepan, combine pomegranate juice, water, and sugar. Bring to a boil, then reduce the heat and simmer for 5 minutes.
2. Remove from heat and let the cordial cool before using.

# THYME SYRUP

## Ingredients

- 1 cup water
- 1 cup granulated sugar
- 5 sprigs fresh thyme

## Procedure

1. In a saucepan, combine water, sugar, and thyme sprigs. Bring to a boil, then reduce the heat and simmer for 5 minutes.
2. Remove from heat and let the mixture steep for 15 minutes.
3. Strain out the thyme and let the infusion cool before using.

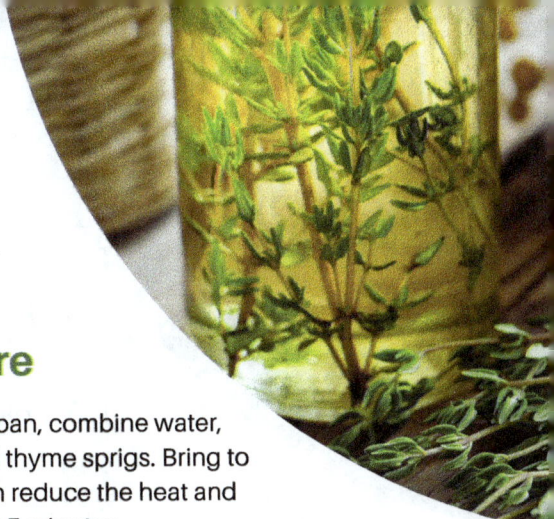

# COCONUT SYRUP

## Ingredients

- 1 cup water
- 1 cup granulated sugar
- 1/2 cup coconut milk

## Procedure

1. In a saucepan, combine water, sugar, and coconut milk. Bring to a boil, then reduce the heat and simmer for 5 minutes.
2. Remove from heat and let the syrup cool before using.

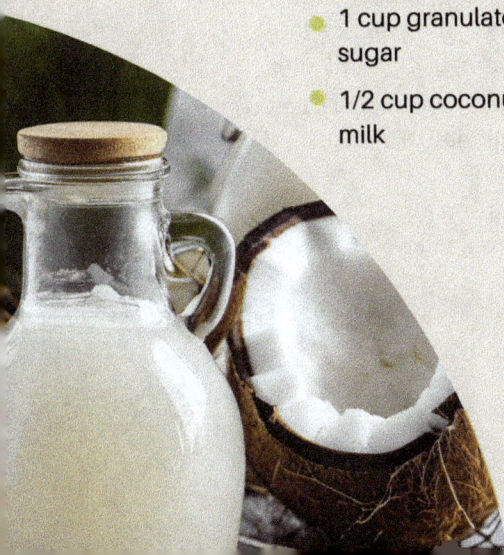

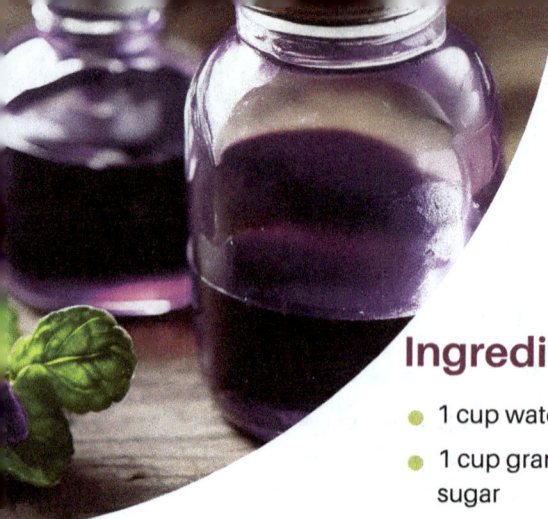

# VIOLET SYRUP

## Ingredients

- 1 cup water
- 1 cup granulated sugar
- 1/2 cup fresh violet flowers (or 1 tablespoon dried, food-grade violet flowers)

## Procedure

1. In a saucepan, combine water, sugar, and violet flowers. Bring to a boil, then reduce the heat and simmer for 5 minutes
2. Remove from heat and let the syrup steep for 15 minutes.
2. Strain out the violet flowers and let the syrup cool before using.

# LEMONGRASS SYRUP

## Ingredients

- 1 cup water
- 1 cup granulated sugar
- 2 stalks fresh lemongrass, chopped

## Procedure

1. In a saucepan, combine water, sugar, and chopped lemongrass. Bring to a boil, then reduce the heat and simmer for 10 minutes.
2. Remove from heat and let it steep for an additional 15 minutes.
3. Strain out the lemongrass and let the syrup cool before using.

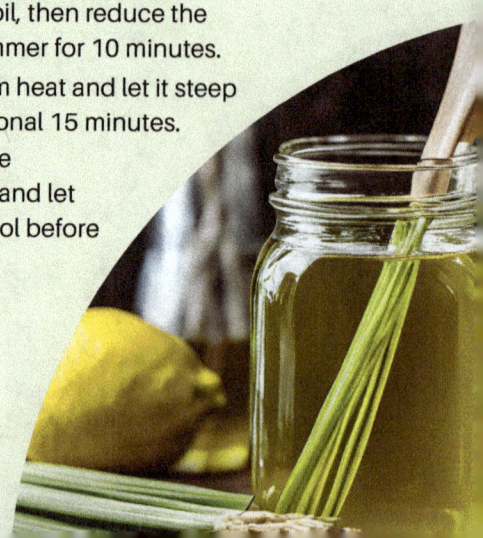

# ROSE SYRUP

## Ingredients

- 1 cup water
- 1 cup granulated sugar
- 1 cup fresh rose petals (or 1 tablespoon dried, food-grade rose petals)

## Procedure

1. In a saucepan, combine water, sugar, and rose petals. Bring to a boil, then reduce the heat and simmer for 5 minutes.
2. Remove from heat and let the syrup steep for 15 minutes.
3. Strain out the rose petals and let the syrup cool before using.

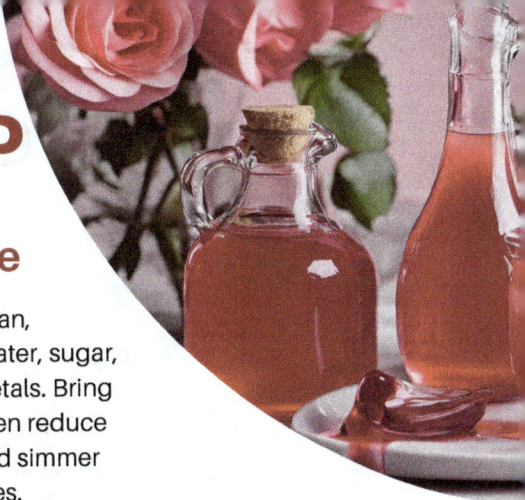

# HONEY SYRUP

## Ingredients

- 1/2 cup honey
- 1/2 cup water

## Procedure

1. In a saucepan, combine honey and water. Heat over low heat, stirring until the honey dissolves completely.
2. Remove from heat and let the syrup cool before using.

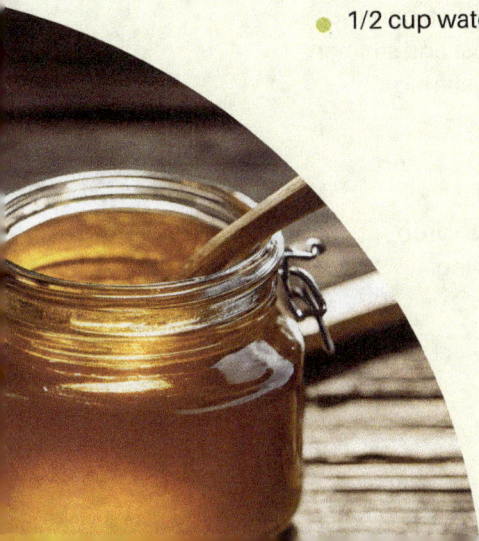

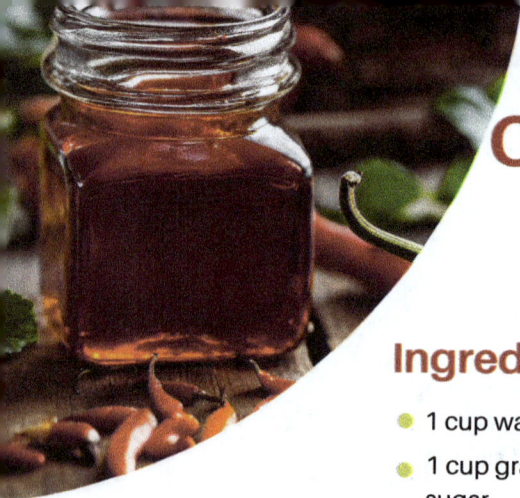

# CHILLI-INFUSED SYRUP

## Ingredients

- 1 cup water
- 1 cup granulated sugar
- 1 fresh chilli pepper, sliced

## Procedure

1. In a saucepan, combine water, sugar, and chilli slices. Bring to a boil, then reduce the heat and simmer for 5 minutes.
2. Remove from heat and let the syrup steep for 15 minutes.
3. Strain out the chilli slices and let the syrup cool before using.

# CHOCOLATE SYRUP

## Ingredients

- 1 cup water
- 1 cup granulated sugar
- 1/2 cup cocoa powder
- 1 teaspoon vanilla extract

## Procedure

1. In a saucepan, combine water, sugar, and cocoa powder. Bring to a boil, then reduce the heat and simmer for 5 minutes, stirring constantly.
2. Remove from heat and stir in the vanilla extract. Let the syrup cool before using.

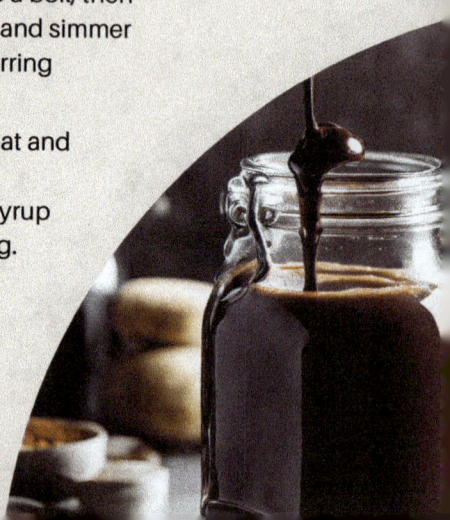

# SPICED CLOVE SYRUP

## Ingredients

- 1 cup water
- 1 cup granulated sugar
- 1 tablespoon whole cloves

## Procedure

1. In a saucepan, combine water, sugar, and mint leaves. Bring to a boil, then reduce the heat and simmer for 5 minutes.
2. Remove from heat and let the syrup steep for 15 minutes.
3. Strain out the cloves and let the syrup cool before using.

# VANILLA BEAN SYRUP

## Ingredients

- 1 cup water
- 1 cup granulated sugar
- 1 vanilla bean, split

## Procedure

1. In a saucepan, combine water, sugar, and the split vanilla bean. Bring to a boil, then reduce the heat and simmer for 5 minutes.
2. Remove from heat and let the syrup steep for 15 minutes.
3. Remove the vanilla bean and let the syrup cool before using.

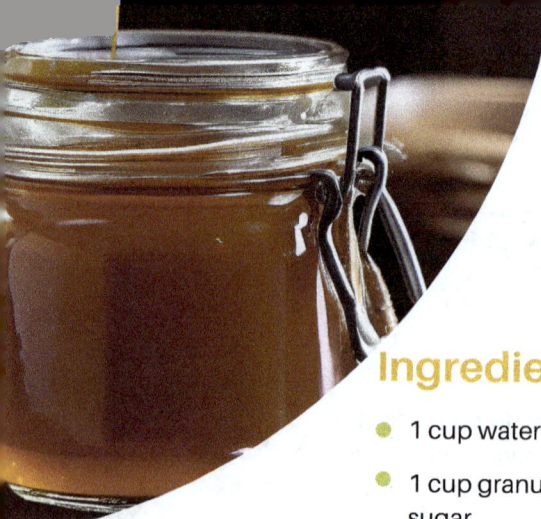

# CARAMEL SYRUP

## Ingredients

- 1 cup water
- 1 cup granulated sugar
- 1/2 cup brown sugar
- 1/4 cup heavy cream

## Procedure

1. In a saucepan, combine water, granulated sugar, and brown sugar. Bring to a boil, then reduce the heat and simmer for 10 minutes.
2. Remove from heat, then slowly stir in the cream. Let the syrup cool before using.

# DILL INFUSION

## Ingredients

- 1 cup water
- 1 cup granulated sugar
- 1/2 cup fresh dill sprigs

## Procedure

1. In a saucepan, combine water, sugar, and dill sprigs. Bring to a boil, then reduce the heat and simmer for 5 minutes.
2. Remove from heat and let the infusion steep for 15 minutes.
3. Strain out the dill and let the infusion cool before using.

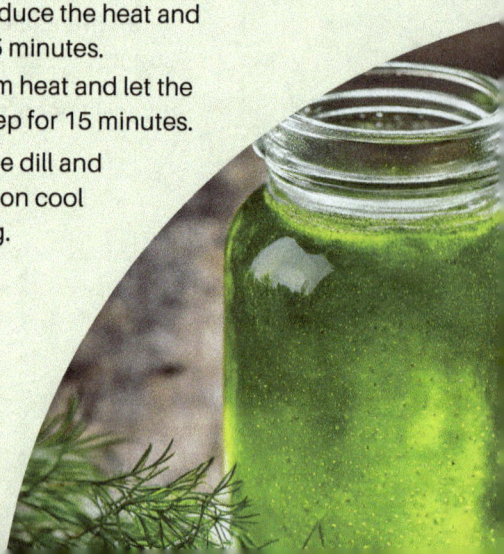

Thank you for choosing *Easy and Delicious MOCKTAILS for Every Day!* We hope this book inspires you to shake, stir, and sip your way through countless delightful, alcohol-free moments.

 We'd love to know what you think! Your feedback means the world to us and helps us create even better books in the future. Simply scan the QR code below to:

- Leave a review and share your favorite recipes with us!
- Connect with us on social media to join the fun and share your mocktail creations.
- Join our email list for updates on new releases, exclusive content, and special offers.

Let's stay in touch and keep the inspiration flowing!

Cheers to your mocktail adventures,

**The Green Sauce Publishing Team**

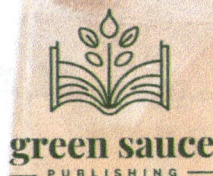

green sauce
— PUBLISHING —

# ALSO AVAILABLE, GET THE WHOLE SERIES!

The Mocktails for Every Day Series is growing! Use the QR Code on page 78 to sign up for notifications so you can be the first to know when the new books are published.

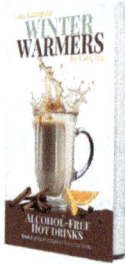

### Cozy & Delightful Winter Warmers

Warm and Cozy, comforting and delicious. Our Winter Warmers are just perfect for long Winter evenings or cozy Winter mornings, or any occasion with friends and family.

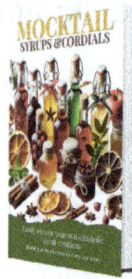

### Mocktail Syrups & Cordials

All our homemade syrups, cordials and infusions gathered together in one beautiful book. Use our syrups in any drinks, or gift them to your friends and family

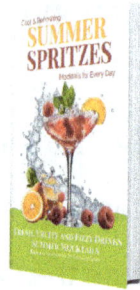

### Cool & Refreshing Summer Spritzes Mocktails for Every Day

Thirst quenching, beautiful and delicious. Our Summer Spritzes are the perfect alcohol-free accompaniment for any occasion, for anyone.

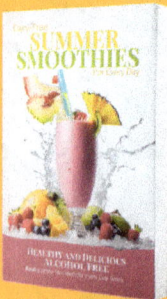

### Dairy-Free Summer Smoothies

Deliciously creamy, but 100% Dairy Free, our Delicious Dairy-Free Summer Smoothies will take your summer mornings to the next level!

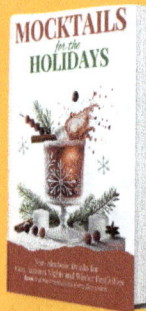

### Mocktails for the Holidays

The ultimate Holiday Mocktail recipe book for any holiday occasion, or just for a fun and festive party for one. A perfect holiday gift too!

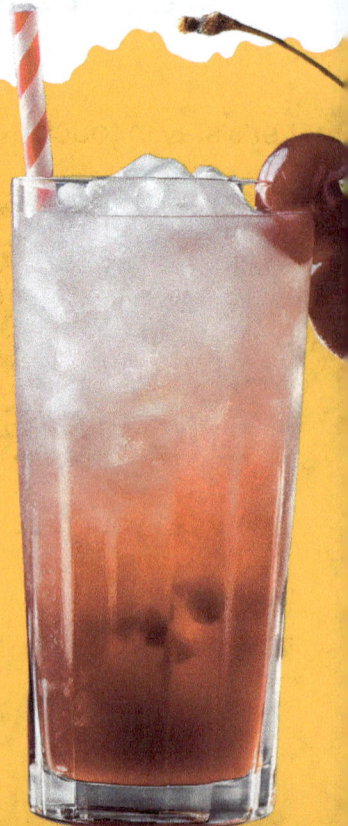